A guide for raising happy, healthy children

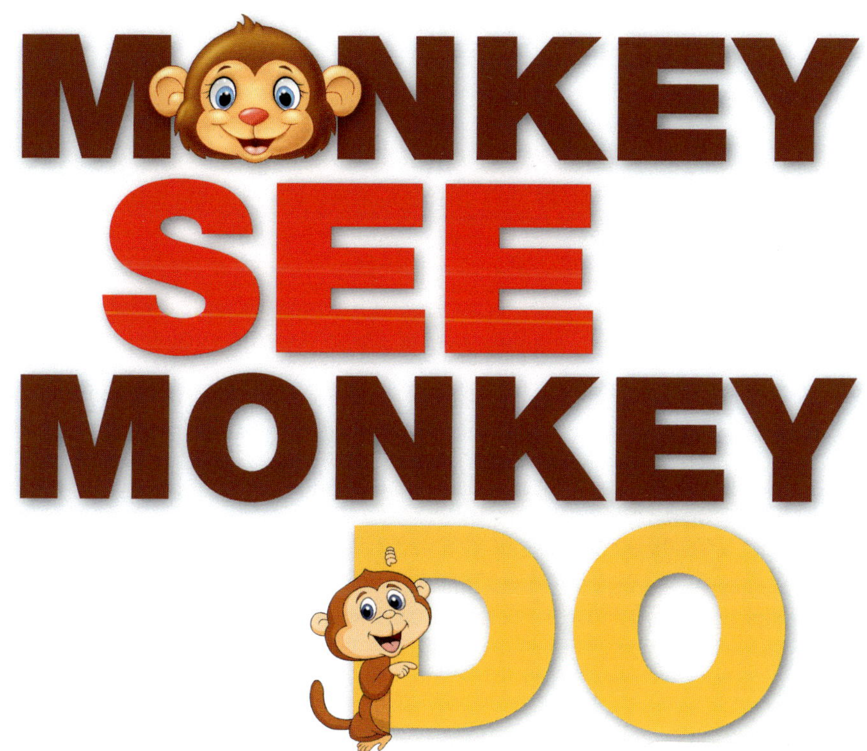

Therese Lemura
Dr Shirley Mcilvenny

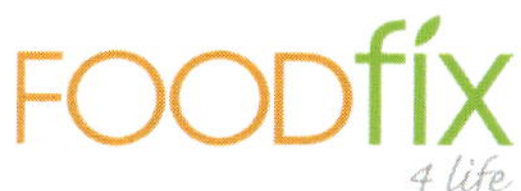

Disclaimer

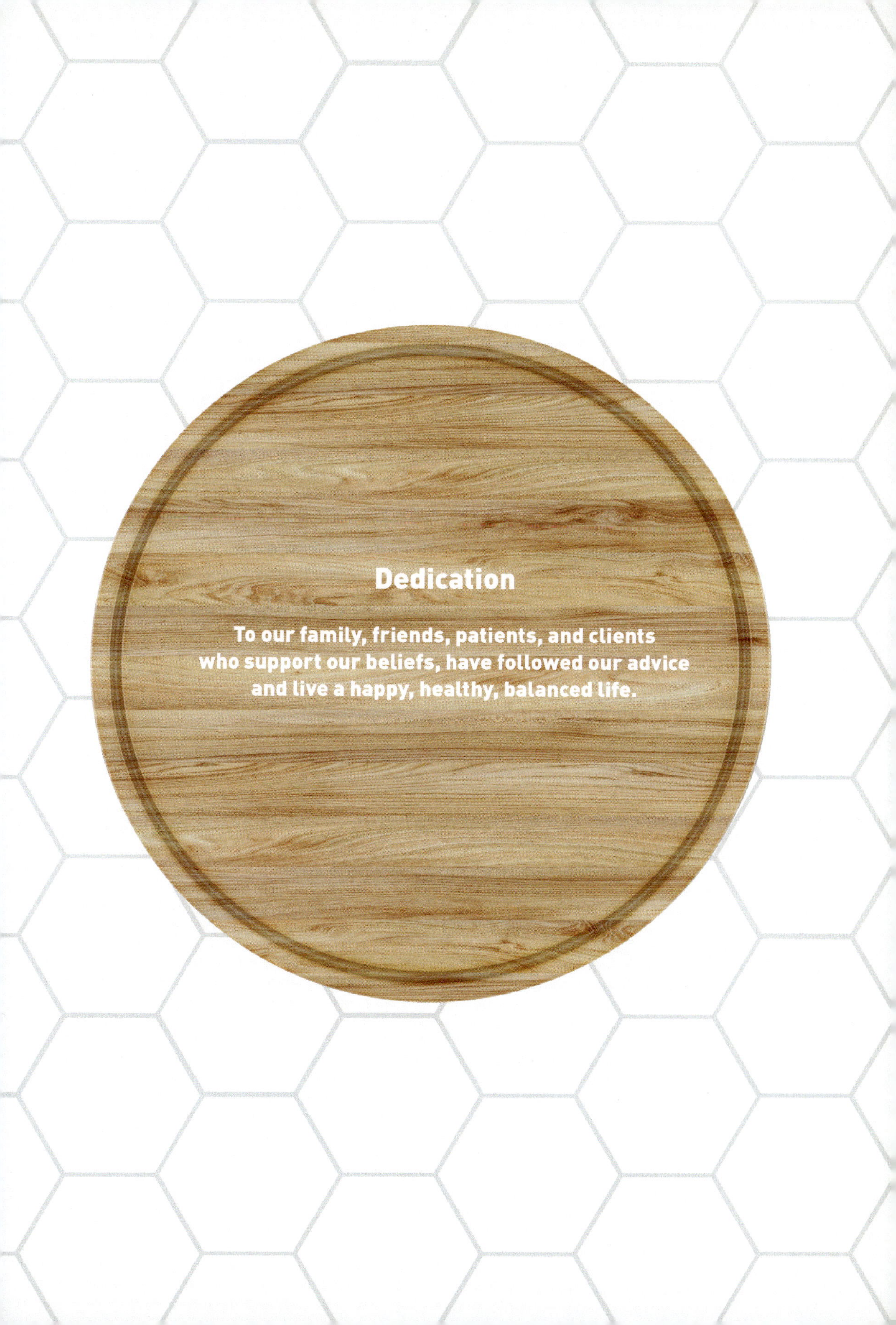

Dedication

To our family, friends, patients, and clients
who support our beliefs, have followed our advice
and live a happy, healthy, balanced life.

Contents

Part 1 For Everyone

Part 2 The specifics

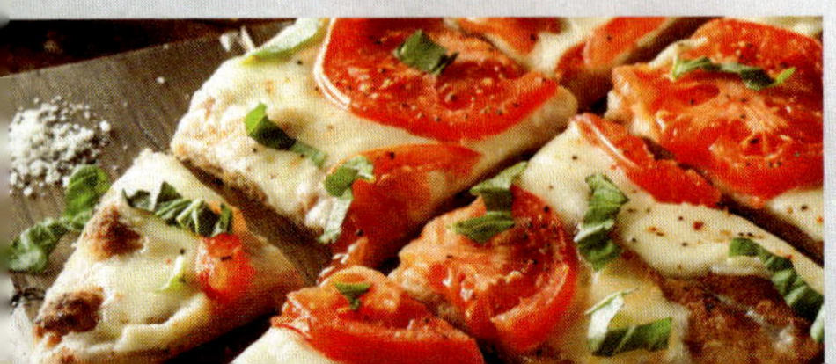
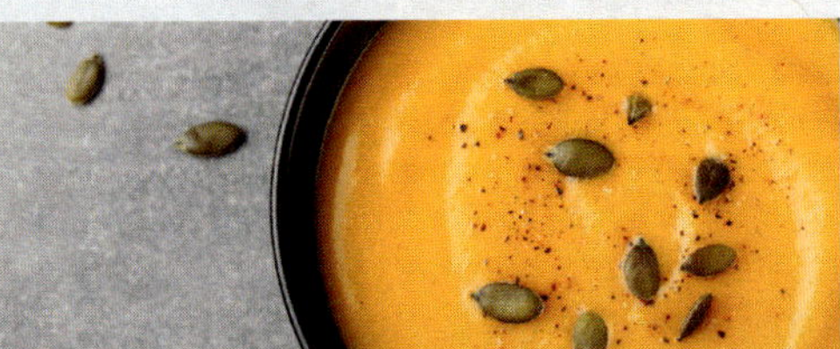
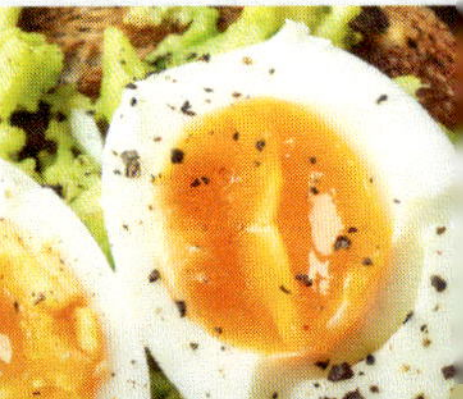

Part 3 Back to school, after school, and party planning

Part 4 Recipes

Part 5 Family menu plan

Appendix

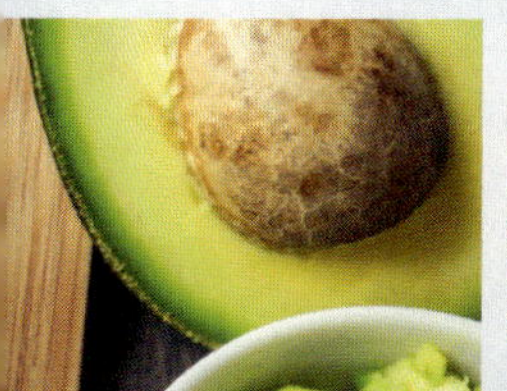
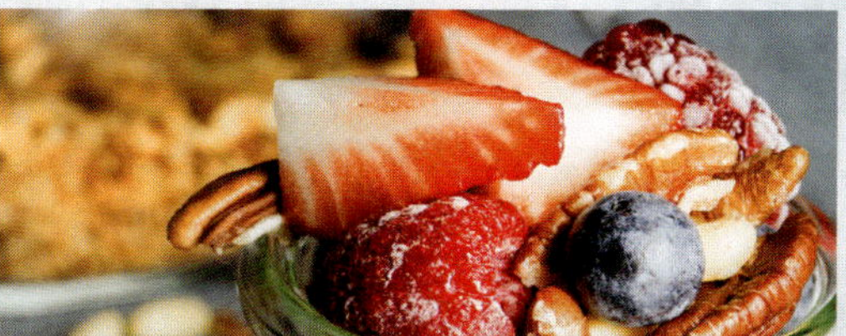
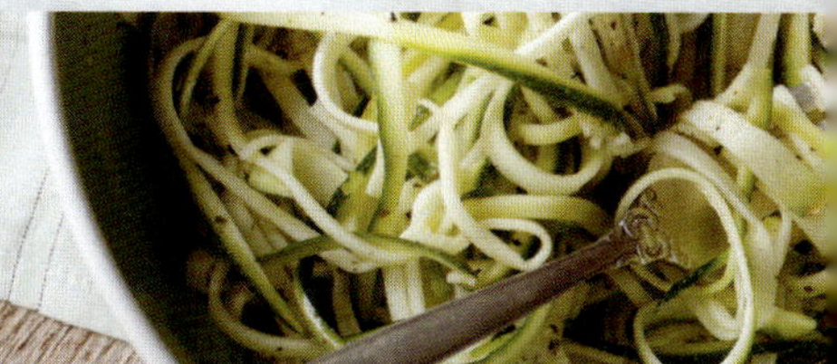

Foreword

This book is based on a simple and practical approach to parenting which encourages laughter and fun while promoting happy, healthy and active children, at home and in the kitchen.

For the parents out there you're not alone. Change will happen, given routine, enthusiasm, and some tender loving care. Watching your children thrive and grow happily is such an achievement. So be proud. If something doesn't work in your household, don't give up, try something else, be persistent. Put your hand up, never be embarrassed to ask for help, and never underestimate the power of being a good role model.

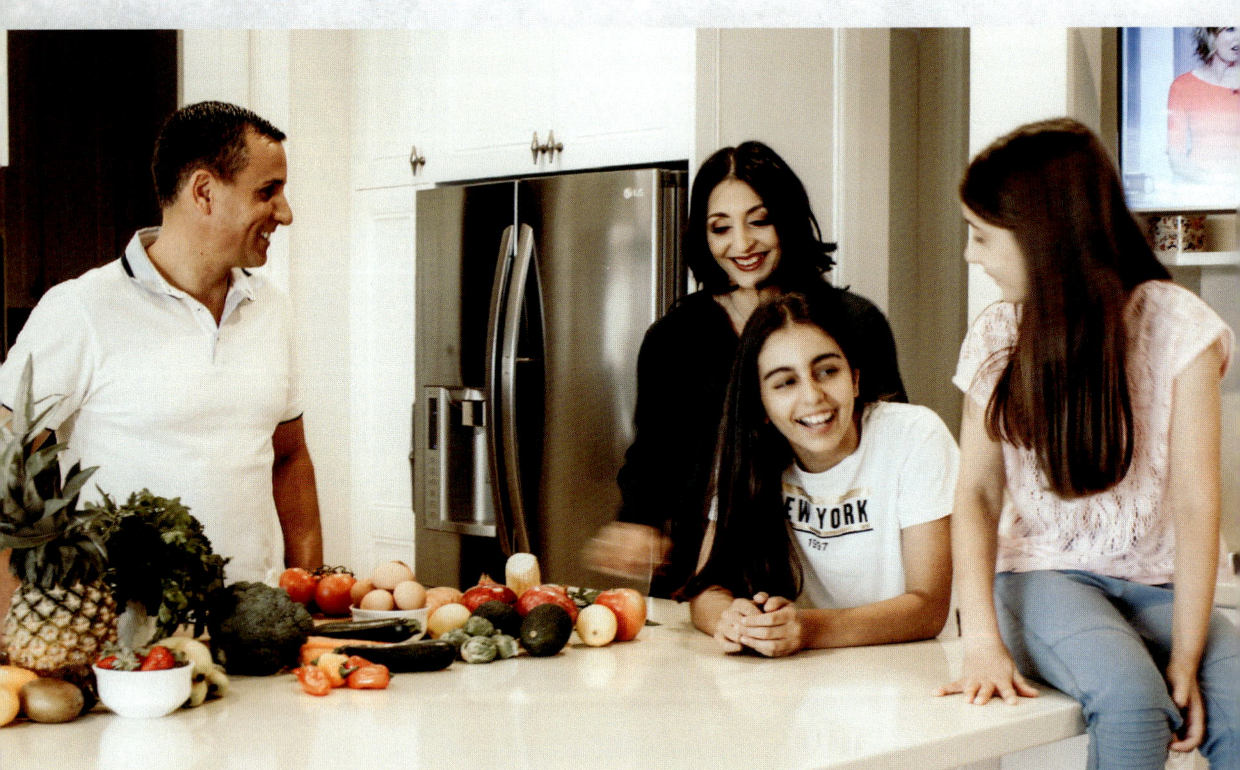

Introduction

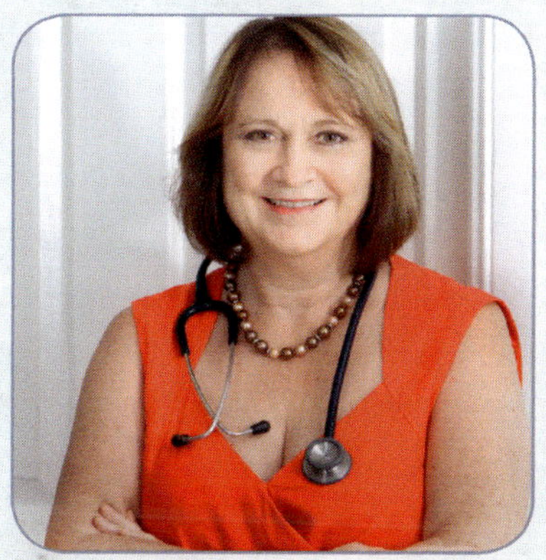

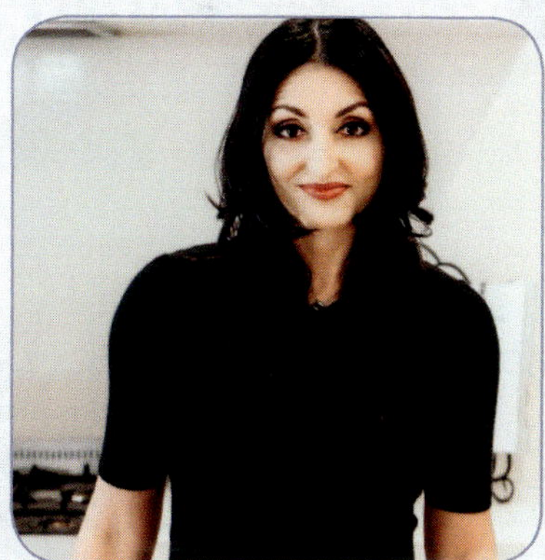

The most important thing you can do as a parent is to feed your children the right diet. Now that may sound easy, but many parents are super busy and lack the time and inspiration to help their kids eat healthily. The aim of this book is to provide information and ideas, and help to make sure your children are getting the best food you can make.

As a busy family doctor, I spend a lot of time helping families become more healthy by changing their diet. For me, it's the one vital thing that will make a huge difference to everyone's health. So dip into this book, use the information, try out some of the recipes and start to enjoy life with your kids more!

– Shirley Mcilvenny

As a parent, finding time to juggle work, family, exercise, cooking, and cleaning has become increasingly difficult. The busy world we live in and expectations of a healthy lifestyle are not as black and white as it seems. No longer is it safe for kids to play alone at the park or even walk to and from school, leaving activity and movement another focus for busy parents. Then there is the biggest focus of all, getting children away from the television or computer screens.

Luckily for my family, healthy meals, the 80/20 rule, saying 'no', and a roster for screen time is a daily occurrence. For most parents, these simple rules do not come easy, so the idea of writing this book to help other families began.

Children need to get into the kitchen, get involved, and learn the principles of healthy eating from a young age. They need to explore, experiment, and have some fun along the way. Remember to let your kids be kids!

They also need to be active and get up off the couch. Seeing the success and smiles on kids' faces with my Move and Learn program has been very rewarding.

Move and Learn is a structured time for movement with various forms of exercise and some fun play, followed by a 15 minute learning session with a different fruit and vegetable each week. After each session, the children get to try this fruit and vegetable and, while they are eating, we give them some quick nutritional info.

For some kids, this is the only way they discover a liking for particular fruits and vegetables. I've had countless parents thanking me because no matter what they did, they couldn't get their kids to try anything new. Sometimes all it takes is an outsider!

So to all the other mums and dads out there, remember you are not alone. Parenting is difficult and delivers endless challenges. What I have learnt from years of parenting is that the old saying 'Monkey see monkey do' is more powerful than any other influence.

As a role model for my children, I practice what I preach, with balance and sustainability. I exercise, say no to ice cream (sometimes), and eat well, most of the time. I have rules in my house such as you must have a piece of fruit before any other snack. Bread is limited to two slices a day, and only one high-sugar food such as ice cream each week.

With some simple rules, one day your children will just get it. They make decisions based on the rules you have set and, yes, they begin to make the right choices. I have seen this with my girls, but it took a while, so hang in there!

From a work point of view, my practice at home is how I educate on a daily basis, irrespective of age. I also teach other parents to be strong, firm, patient, and never to use food as a reward. I consider myself a normal mum, although some would not agree. I am rather tough on food choices but I have children's best interests at heart. I am my children's best role model and from the start my goal was to raise happy, healthy, and active children.

– Therese Lemura

About us

You can read about our team and qualifications on our website:

www.foodfix4life.com.au

We are also on Instagram and facebook:

Instagram www.instagram.com/foodfix4life

Facebook www.facebook.com/foodfix4life

Jessica Sheargold, Sydney Franchisee

"My love of fresh and real food was inspired by the example that my mother and grandmother set during my upbringing. Being included in the food journey from garden to kitchen to the table has been essential in the food habits I formed early in life, and the skills and understanding I have now."

Susan Bown, Queensland Franchisee

"I was a very stubborn and fussy eater as a child, and remember times I visited friends' houses and ate things I would never eat at home, just because others were. As a teenager and young adult, this became even more of a pattern in trying and accepting new foods. That's why I believe it's important we don't overlook the importance of the social influences on what we eat. Whether at childcare, the family dinner table or while dining out, each experience gives children and adults new opportunities to learn from observing and imitating others."

Thank you

A special thank you to the team for their contributions to recipe development, testing and photography.

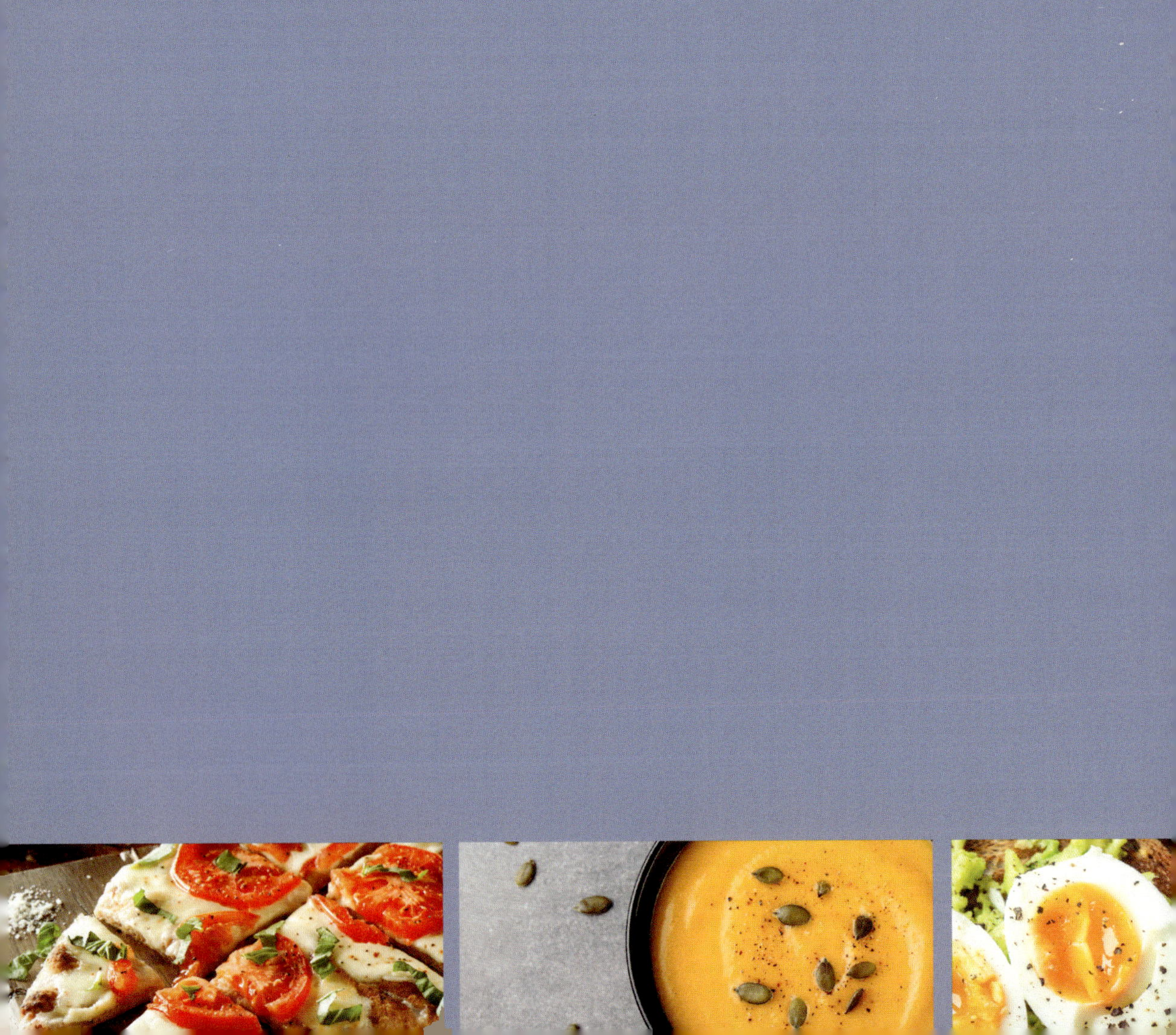

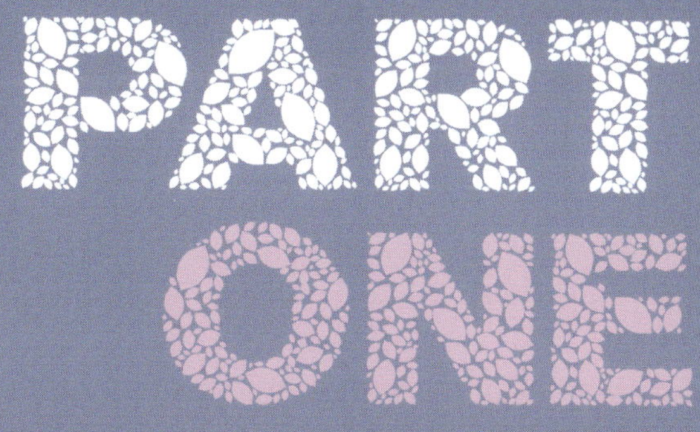

PART ONE

For Everyone

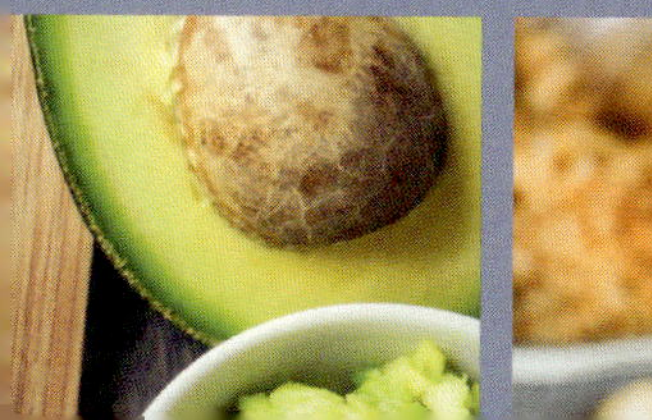
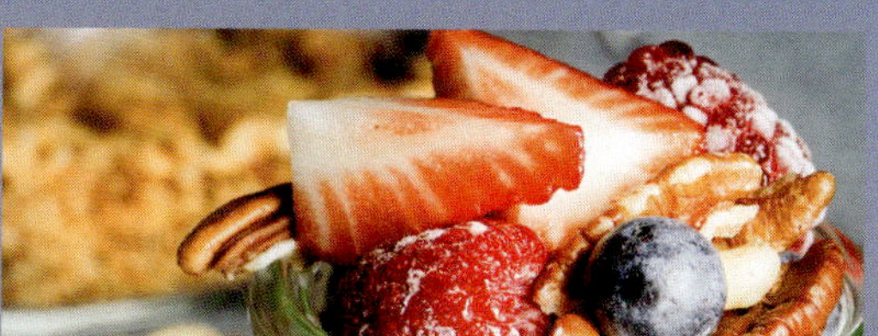
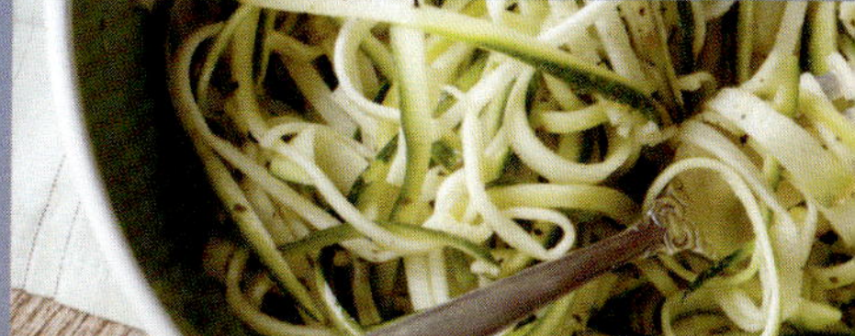

Eating as a family

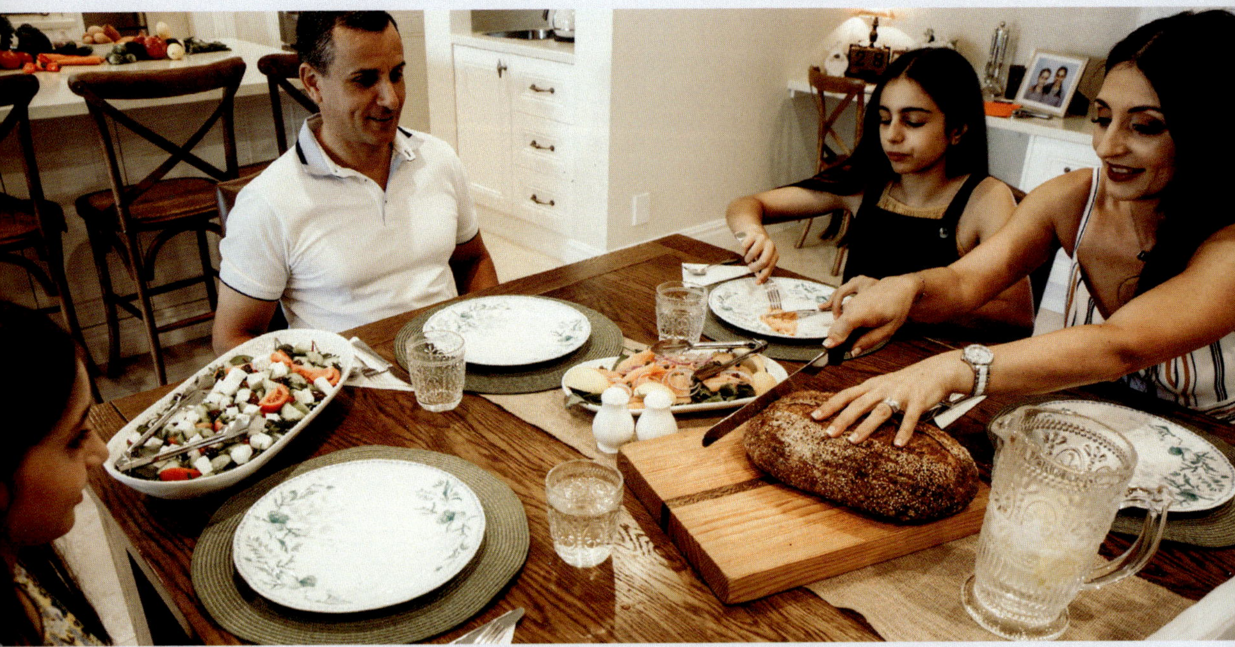

Eating as a family will help your children develop healthy habits early in life that will bring lifelong benefits. Kids will be more likely to try new foods and, as our book title says, *Monkey see monkey do*, they quietly watch what and how much you eat. Family mealtime is an opportunity to provide a role model for healthy eating.

Eating as a family also allows for positive connection and communication. The dinner table is a great way to discuss weekly events, chores and give praise. It should be fun and not a time for disciplinary measures.

As a parent, I also see mealtime as an opportunity to monitor children's moods, behaviour and discuss their activities with friends.

Involving the kids in dinner preparation gets them into the kitchen. They can watch, help and even give cooking a try! This might mean more mess, but it's all part of the learning experience. Teach them how and why you do things the way you do. Pass on those traditional recipes so they can be enjoyed for generations.

When practice becomes a habit

Eventually, all those new ways of eating become a habit and fit naturally into your lifestyle. Without you knowing it, your shopping list has changed, so has what you keep in your fridge, pantry, and ultimately what you cook.

Kids like structure and consistency. The repeat process gives them a sense of security and belonging.

TIPS

- Try the easy recipes in this book.
- Find a food coach to help you plan meals while incorporating your likes, dislikes and lifestyle.
- Use the internet to save shopping time.
- Try farmers markets for fresh and cheaper produce.

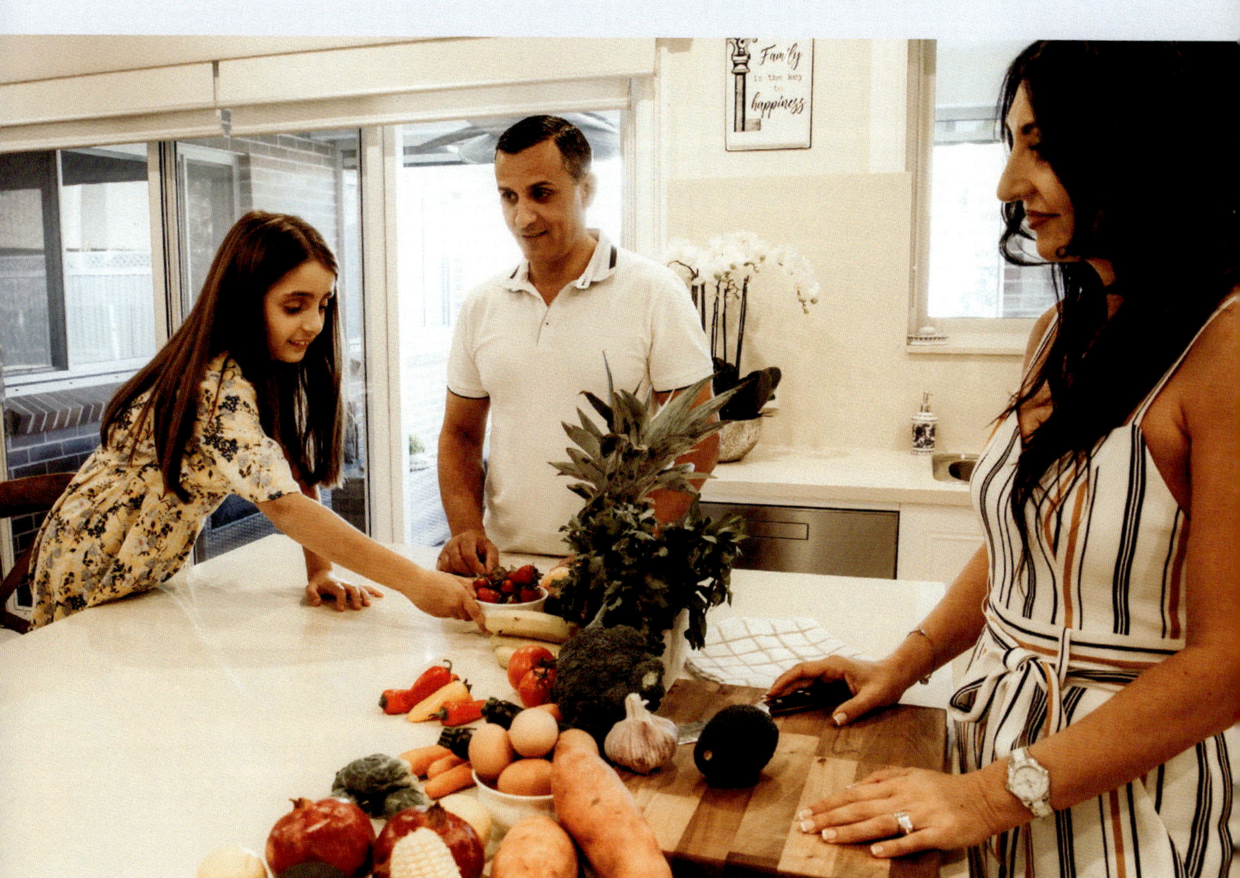

From paddock to plate

In Australia, the Paddock to Plate movement emphasises quality, promotes fresh is best, and it leaves behind packaged convenience foods.

Many of us do not understand that most -packaged supermarket foods are processed and contain preservatives, artificial sweeteners, flavourings and colourings.

So how do we get maximum nutrients from the food we eat? Simple, eat fresh!

When you grow your own produce, it is picked as needed when it is ripe and bursting with nutrients. It requires no preservatives or additives to extend shelf life. Your menu should always be based on seasonality.

What can we do to make healthier choices?

There are many things we can do to reduce our families' exposure to artificial chemicals in food. As consumers we are more powerful than we imagine and can have a big influence on supermarkets and food producers. Shops are now selling much more gluten-free produce because lots of people are looking for these products. Organic markets are also springing up.

Start by preparing meals that are made with fresh food rather than processed products. That gets rid of preservatives, flavourings and colourings straight off. Then try to buy organic whenever you can – that includes meat, vegetables and fruit.

Many people say they can't afford organic food. In that case, try buying organic versions of vegetables and fruit such as broccoli, celery and strawberries that we know are sprayed many times with pesticides.

TIP

Buy from local growers, farms direct and growers markets.

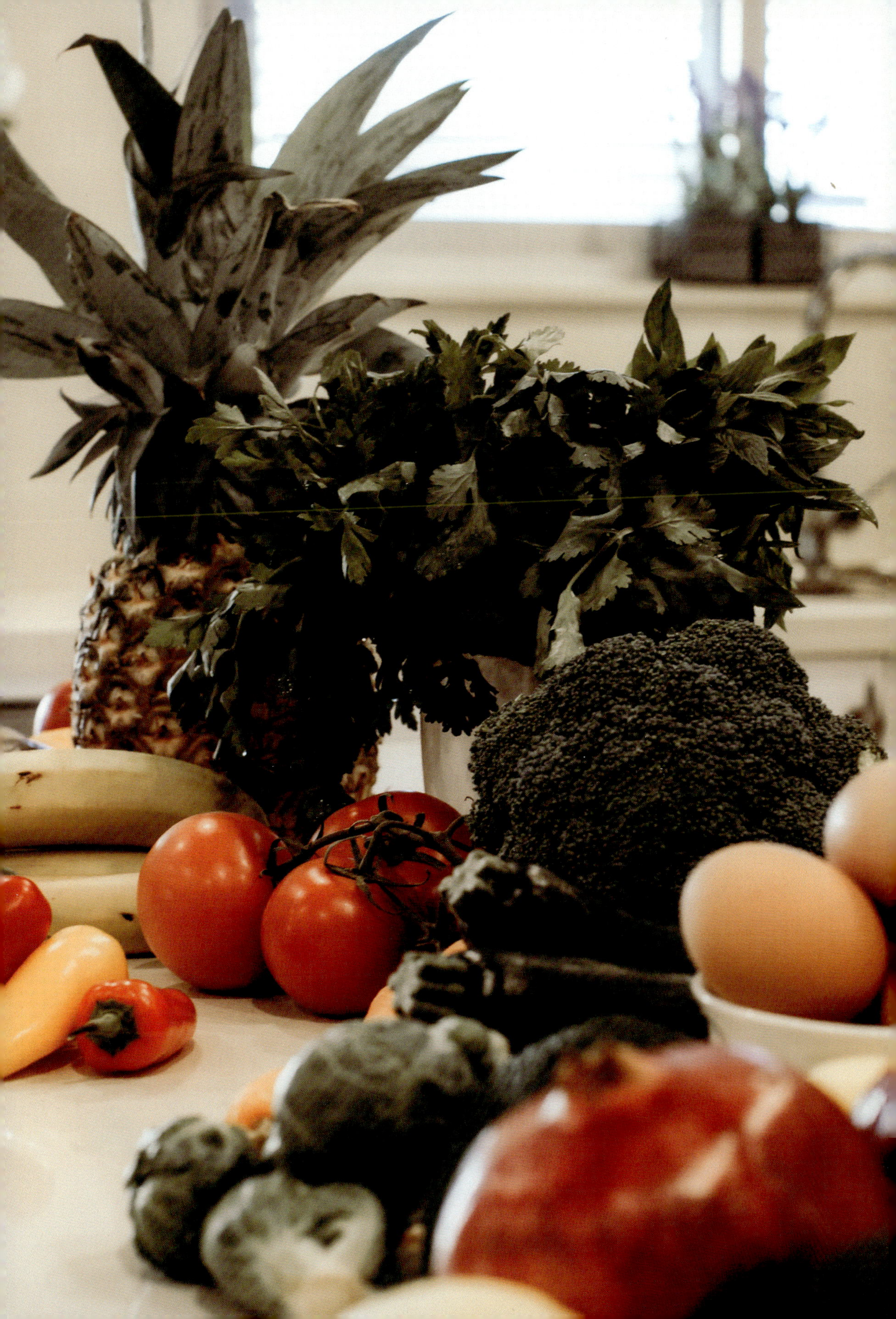

Teaching kids balance and portion control

This is a big pitfall in many households. We simply eat too much.

The amount we eat is as dependent on physical activity levels as it is on the way we have learnt to eat.

Teaching children from an early age is crucial. Particular foods may be limited sometimes, dessert is not necessary every night, and the importance of fruit and vegetables is the way to go.

Teach them to balance out their day. If they are eating dinner out, do they need a day full of snacks? Try on these days to have only breakfast and lunch with no snacks.

Serving size versus portion size

There is a difference and, yes, it matters:

- Serving size is found on the nutritional label and is what the manufacturer *suggests*.
- Portion size is the amount of a food you choose to eat at any one time, which may be more or less than a serving.

Some rules to try in your household are

- A maximum of two slices of bread a day.
- One to two serves of fruit before any snack.
- Eat only at specified meal times such as breakfast, morning tea, lunch, afternoon tea, and dinner.
- One packaged snack a day, if necessary.
- Dessert once a week.
- One serve each of milk and/or yoghurt a day.
- If having a meal out, make other meals lighter and low in carbohydrates.

Serve size examples

- A teaspoon of butter is the size of one dice.
- Generally a serve of meat is the size of a deck of cards.
- A serve of cheese is the size of four stacked dice.
- One slice of bread is one serve.
- ½ cup rice or pasta (cooked) is a serve.
- One small piece of fruit (super-large apples are two + servings) is a serve.
- One wedge of melon is a serve.

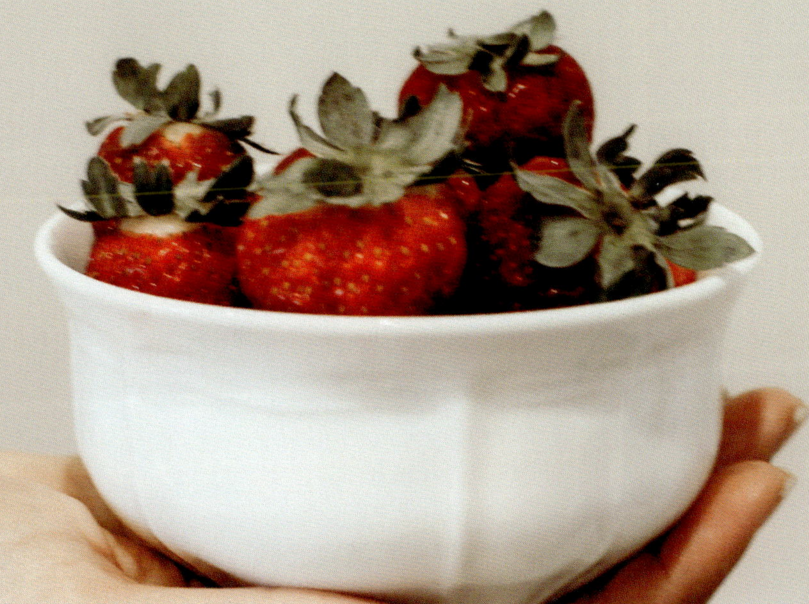

TIPS

- Do not skip meals.
- If unsure, measure and weigh food for a week to visually understand how much is required.
- Learn good eating out habits. Choose healthier options and always include salad or vegetables. Learn how to compromise with tempting breads and desserts.
- Try using a smaller dinner plate.
- Seconds should be a little more protein, salad or vegetables.
- Always eat from a plate.
- Buy 'portion perfection' plates for the family to try.
- Invest in a single consultation with your nutrition coach to have a meal plan tailored to your portion-specific needs. This way you can ensure you get all your necessary macro and micronutrients each day.

Fussy eaters

Many children are fussy eaters. We have all heard about one of these. Having one is another story as they can be hard to handle.

All kids have their moments, however it's not forever. Their eating habits change. We need to be consistent, patient and constantly educate on all things healthy and not.

It's normal for children not to like the shape, colour or texture of particular foods. It's also normal for children to like something one day but dislike it the next, to refuse to try new foods, and to eat more or less, from day to day. The good news is that children are likely to get less fussy as they get older.

If you have major concerns about your child's growth and development, please see your doctor or nutritionist for help and assessment.

Tips for handling fussy eaters

- Make mealtimes routine and about happy, family time.
- Praise your child for any small effort to try a new food.
- Never force your child to try a food.
- Make healthy foods fun, e.g., cut sandwiches into interesting shapes.
- Let your child help prepare a salad or whisk the eggs for an omelette.
- Children are likely to mimic the eating habits of their parents – *monkey see monkey do*, so set a good example!
- Kids have small stomachs, so small and frequent meals are best.
- Variety will help – make simple but different recipes with the basics.
- No juice, water only.
- For most foods there is almost always a substitute:
  - if they don't like milk, try cheese.
  - if they don't like chewing chicken, try chicken mince.
- Reintroduce foods they don't like on a regular basis.
- When kids are unwell, they will want only certain foods in small quantities.
- Stay positive, try not to yell and get upset.

Activity and movement

Regular physical activity and movement skills are a building block for a young child's healthy and active life.

If habits are developed early, children are more likely to continue them long term, which will give them excellent foundations for good health and wellbeing. Kids and teens are strongly influenced by role models such as their parents, older siblings, family, friends and teachers. So it is important that while some activity may be planned and structured, some also needs to be fun and improvised.

If a child/teen is not physically active enough, they will not have the chance to adequately develop these skills and good habits and so are at increased risk of becoming overweight or even obese. Long term, being overweight or obese can contribute to conditions such as high blood pressure and cholesterol, type II diabetes and liver disease.

At home there are many ways to get kids moving with minimal equipment, such as:

- Ball games in the yard
- Balloon tennis
- Table tennis
- Basketball
- Elastics
- Skipping
- Hide and seek.

This sort of play gets them off the couch and away from screens.

Something a little more structured may be at the park when they can have running or climbing races. Free play is a must too, as it is fun and lets kids be kids!

Starting them early in sport is great for developing confidence, team play and discipline. Among the options here are little athletics, soccer, dancing, tennis, netball etc.

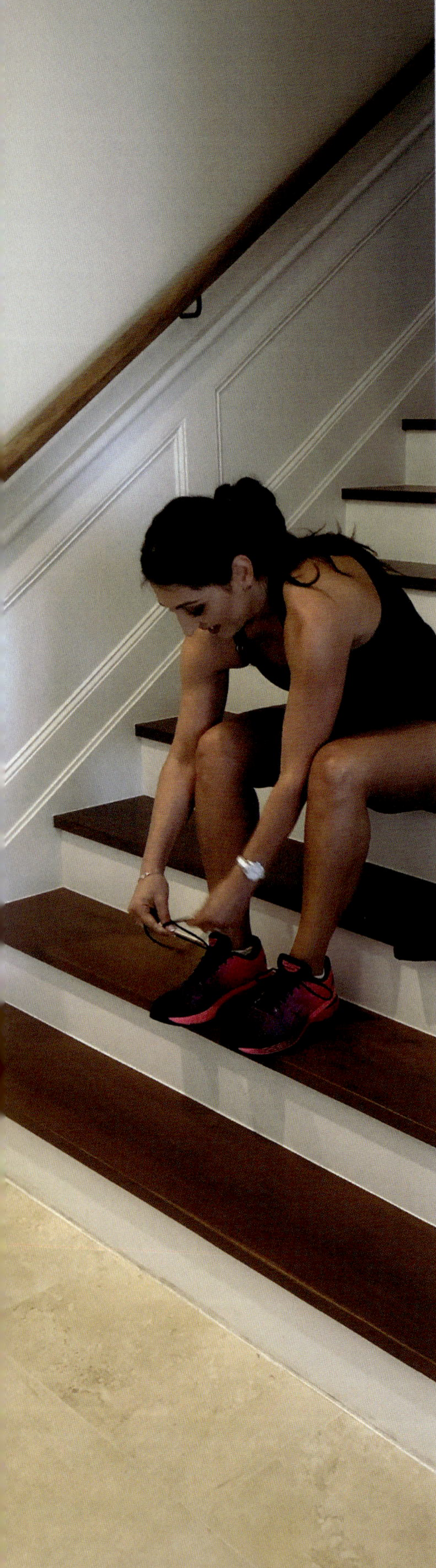

At school children get to try a variety of sports they may wish to take up as an after-school competitive sport.

As kids move into their teens, there is generally a sport they would like to play.

How much is needed?

- Incidental movement at home, away from the couch should be at least 30 minutes a day.
- Activity where the heart rate is elevated at least three times a week.
- For weight loss this needs to be five times a week.
- Most teenagers/adults should be doing 30 minutes a day, four to five times a week. This should include weight bearing exercises as well as structured activity.

Benefits of activity and movement for all ages

- Promotes growth and development of bones, muscles, flexibility and balance.
- Helps achieve and maintain a healthy weight.
- Improves confidence and self-esteem.
- Develops social skills.
- Improves cardiovascular fitness.

What can I do to help my children be active?

- Be an active role model. Let your children see what physical activity you enjoy.
- Encourage active play in the backyard, go for a fast walk, dance to music, ride a bike or engage in more vigorous activities such as running and swimming.
- Make time to be active as a family – walk to the shops, school or the park. Try bike riding or walking the dog.
- Limit screen time.

Fun facts

- Screen time for fun, not education, is linked to kids and teens becoming overweight.
- Those who spend more than two hours a day on their screens are less likely to eat healthily and participate in physical activity.
- Those with a more sedentary lifestyle are more likely to choose foods high in sugar, salt and saturated fat.

Remember

- Children should wear appropriate footwear for support.
- Hats and sunscreen are needed for all outdoor play.
- Encourage children to drink plenty of water only, during and after all sport/activity.
- A healthy diet and an active child go hand in hand.
- Learn to say 'no'; get them into the kitchen and limit the sugar and processed foods/drinks.

TIPS

- Try a roster for screen time/park play/structured activity or sport.
- Learn to say 'no'.
- Monitor what they are watching/playing on TV and devices.
- No TV or devices in the bedroom.

Eating for sport

Kids need fuel for growth and development, but also for sport. This is where the energy intake of kids/adolescents goes beyond maintenance, as it needs to meet the demands of daily energy expenditure. The way to calculate this is to listen to your child's needs and combine enough protein, fats and carbohydrate before and after sport.

As parents, we need to set good foundations for nutrition. It is also a good idea to practise what we preach, by making good nutritional choices most of the time. Believe it or not, kids are always watching us.

Good nutrition:

- Promotes energy
- Prevents fatigue, injury and disease
- Improves strength, speed and endurance
- Maintains a healthy weight

How do we do it?

- With foods that are good sources of energy
- Eating at the right time of day
- Eating before, during and after sport

Macros – carbohydrate, protein and fat

Recommendations for carbohydrate, protein and fat intake depend on the activity/sport load.

Combining a carb and protein will help recovery after training/competition.

Fat needs to come from healthy unsaturated fats such as olive oil, avocado, nuts and seeds and no more than 10 per cent of total daily energy coming from saturated fats.

Macronutrients needed for energy

	Benefits	Good sources
Carbohydrates	Provide glucose needed for energy	Whole grains, vegetables, fruits, milk and yoghurt
Protein	Builds and repairs muscle, hair, nails and skin Helps maintain glucose when doing physical activity for long periods	Lean meat and poultry, fish, eggs, dairy products, beans and nuts
Fats	Help the body absorb vitamins A, D, E and K; protect the body's organs and provide insulation	Lean meat and poultry, fish, nuts, seeds, dairy products and olive oil Fat from chips, fried foods and baked goods should be minimal.

Micronutrients

Many vitamins and minerals are required for good health. Consuming particular nutrients such as calcium, Vitamin D and iron should be monitored. Calcium is important for bone health, normal enzyme activity and muscle contraction. Calcium is found in a variety of foods and beverages, including milk, yoghurt, cheese, broccoli, spinach and fortified grain products.

Vitamin D is necessary for bone health and to absorb calcium. Some sources of Vitamin D include salmon, eggs, mushrooms and sunshine.

Iron is important for oxygen delivery to body tissues. During adolescence, more iron is needed to support growth and lean muscle mass. Iron-rich foods include eggs, leafy green vegetables, fortified whole grains and lean meat.

Eating before sport/activity

Meals should include carbohydrates, protein and fat. Fibre should be limited. High-fat meals should be avoided before exercise because they can make you feel sluggish and therefore affect performance. Eating should ideally be one to two hours before sport. If sport is early in the morning try a small snack, a good dinner the night before and a bigger meal after training.

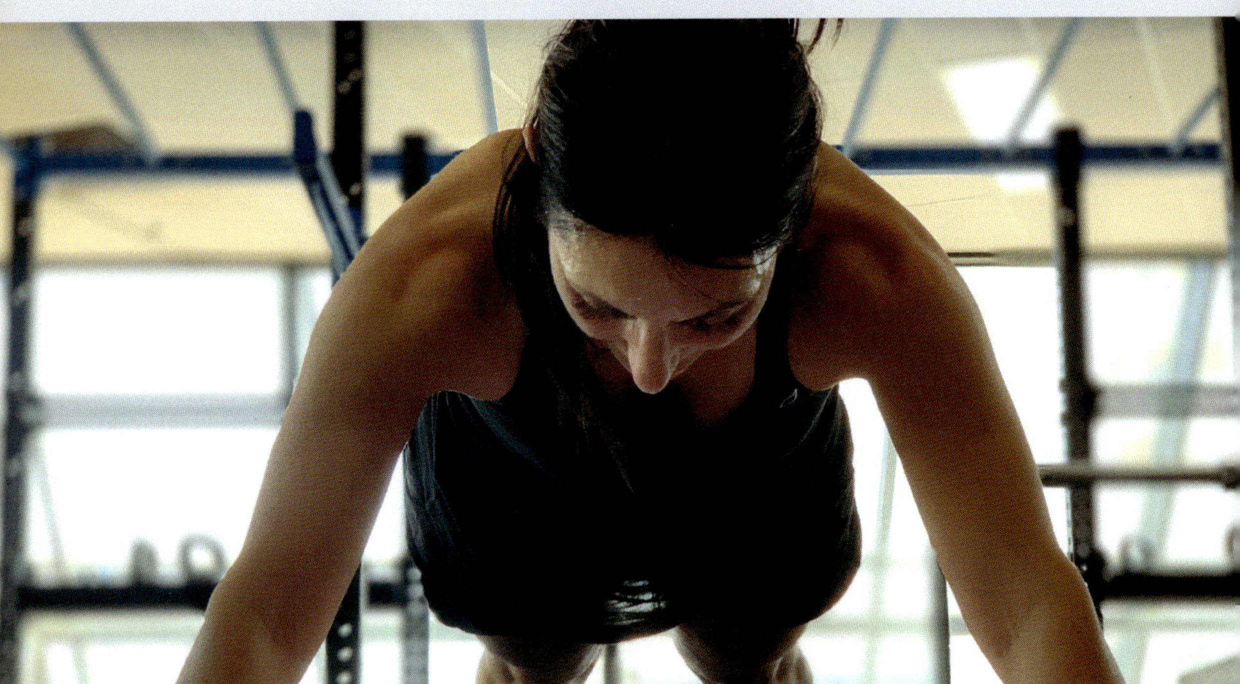

Eating after sport/activity

Foods should be consumed within 30 minutes of exercise to help reload muscles with glycogen and allow for proper recovery. These foods should include protein and carbohydrates.

Meal planning

The timing of meals is very important and needs to be individualised along with food likes/dislikes. See your nutritionist for help with a plan based on activity levels, training and competition.

Fluid for sport

Kids and adolescents should be encouraged to be well hydrated before exercise, particularly in hot environments. Water is needed before, during and after physical activity.

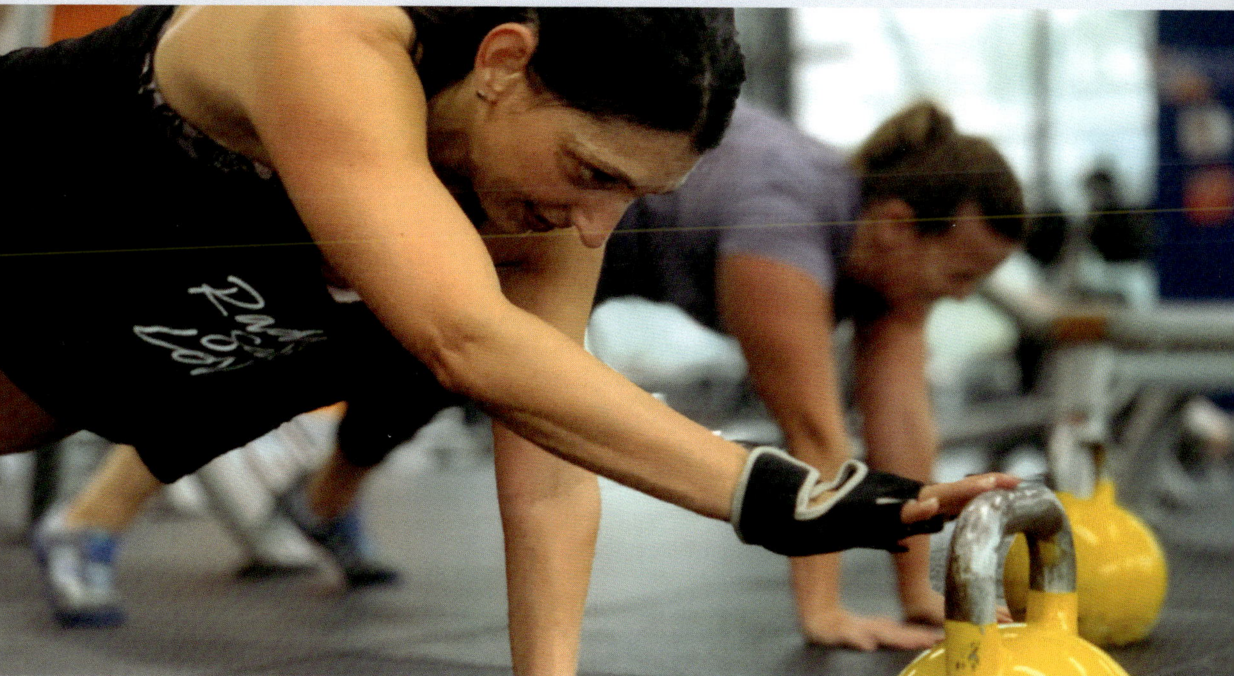

A sports drink?

For the active child/adolescent water is the only beverage needed. Sports drinks instead of water are really not necessary and may lead to excessive caloric consumption. For the highly active/competitive child/adolescent, a sports drink during prolonged vigorous exercise can be beneficial by providing carbohydrate, fluid and electrolytes.

Energy drinks?

These are not the same as a sports drink. Energy drinks are usually highly caffeinated drinks with sugar and not needed at all.

Saying 'no'

As a parent saying 'no' seems to be a daily occurrence.

We all know that giving in is the easier option as it saves the yelling and tantrums. We need to be firm but fair and consistent. Kids will test the waters and it's OK sometimes to give in, but generally we must stay true to our original objective of raising healthy children. They need to be educated with food choices and, if needed, parents should explain their reasoning as they go.

As a parent we call this tough love! If we continue with our tough love we will promote the foundations of our child's eating roadmap.

It is ultimately up to us to decide what foods come into the house, are prepared, and served.

Be parent savvy and determine whether your child is really hungry or just craving food. They are two different responses. Hunger is physiological – a drop in blood sugar level; craving is psychological – due to boredom or emotions.

My advice is to stick to structured eating times, for example, breakfast, morning tea, lunch, afternoon tea, and dinner, as much as possible.

How to say 'no' example:

Child: Can I have a piece of toast?

Mum: No, because you have already had two slices today.

Food labels

Learn to read food labels so you can accurately assess if the snack food is approved or a 'sometimes' food. Let's look at food labels:

1. The ingredients are listed in weight order. If sugar or any form of sugar is number 1, 2 or 3, it belongs back on the shelf. The only exception is where the sugars are naturally occurring, such as in dairy products.

2. Sugar per serve, saturated fat and sodium should be looked at next.

   As a rule of thumb:

   - 5 grams or less of sugar per serve is acceptable
   - 6-8 grams is OK occasionally
   - 8 grams or more is a treat or indulgence.

3. Sodium 120 milligrams or less is low sodium. We do not want or need any more than 1600mg of sodium daily.

4. Saturated fat should never be more than half of the total fat per serve.

   Total saturated fat should not exceed 10g a day.

TIP

Remember, let kids be kids, and the 80/20 rule.

Rest, repair and recharge

We all know the benefits of eating well and exercising, but to repeat this on a daily basis, do we know how to rest, replenish and recover?

Research is finding relaxation has many positive benefits for our health, such as releasing muscle tension, lowering blood pressure, heart rate and cortisol levels.

Types of relaxation techniques include

- Walking outside in the fresh air
- Sitting quietly without the television, phones or radio on
- Yoga
- Meditation
- Massage
- Cat naps.

Long-term relaxation techniques promote better sleep patterns and a stronger immune system.

Relaxation is simply mental gymnastics. Finding just 10 minutes a day for four weeks consistently has proven results such as less anxiety and a more positive mood.

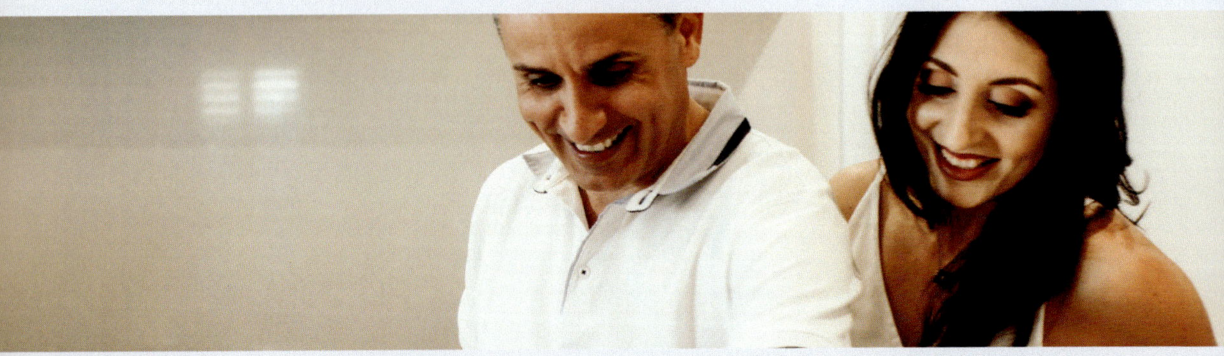

Laughter is good medicine

Sometimes it's the simple things such as laughter that can lower stress levels and boost our immunity. A relaxing environment with laughter and rest is a perfect way to recharge the batteries.

Better sleep

Sleep is a vitally important component of a healthy lifestyle. Most adults need six to eight hours' sleep a night. Children need a lot more. Many people do not get enough sleep and build up a significant sleep debt. Eventually, that debt has to be paid off and people find themselves needing all weekend to recover from work or unable to do anything apart from work and housework.

Health problems associated with lack of sleep

Denying yourself the correct amount of sleep has serious health consequences. We know that lack of sleep affects your memory, your ability to think and to make decisions as well as your co-ordination. This makes you more likely to have a car accident or injury at work.

Poor sleep can increase your appetite by making you crave carbohydrates (to gain more energy). It also lowers leptin, the hormone that controls appetite. So chronic sleep debt can lead to weight gain. Poor sleep is also associated with insulin resistance, which makes us more likely to get diabetes. At the same time, lack of sleep weakens your immune system, making you more vulnerable to colds and flu. People who get too little sleep often age more quickly as their growth hormone production is decreased.

Normal sleep

During the evening, your sleep hormone melatonin increases to prepare you for sleep. Your 24-hour cycle of cortisol, which gives you energy during the day, and melatonin which controls sleep at night, is called the circadian rhythm. Sleep has several stages, such as rapid eye movement (REM) sleep during which you dream. Anything that reduces the amount of REM sleep leads to sleep deprivation. Catching up on REM sleep often results in nightmares during dream cycles.

What is poor sleep?

People have several problems with sleep. One of the most common is difficulty falling asleep. This is often caused by worry and stress. Another common problem is waking during the night and not going back to sleep. Again worry and stress can cause this. Depression can lead to waking early in the morning.

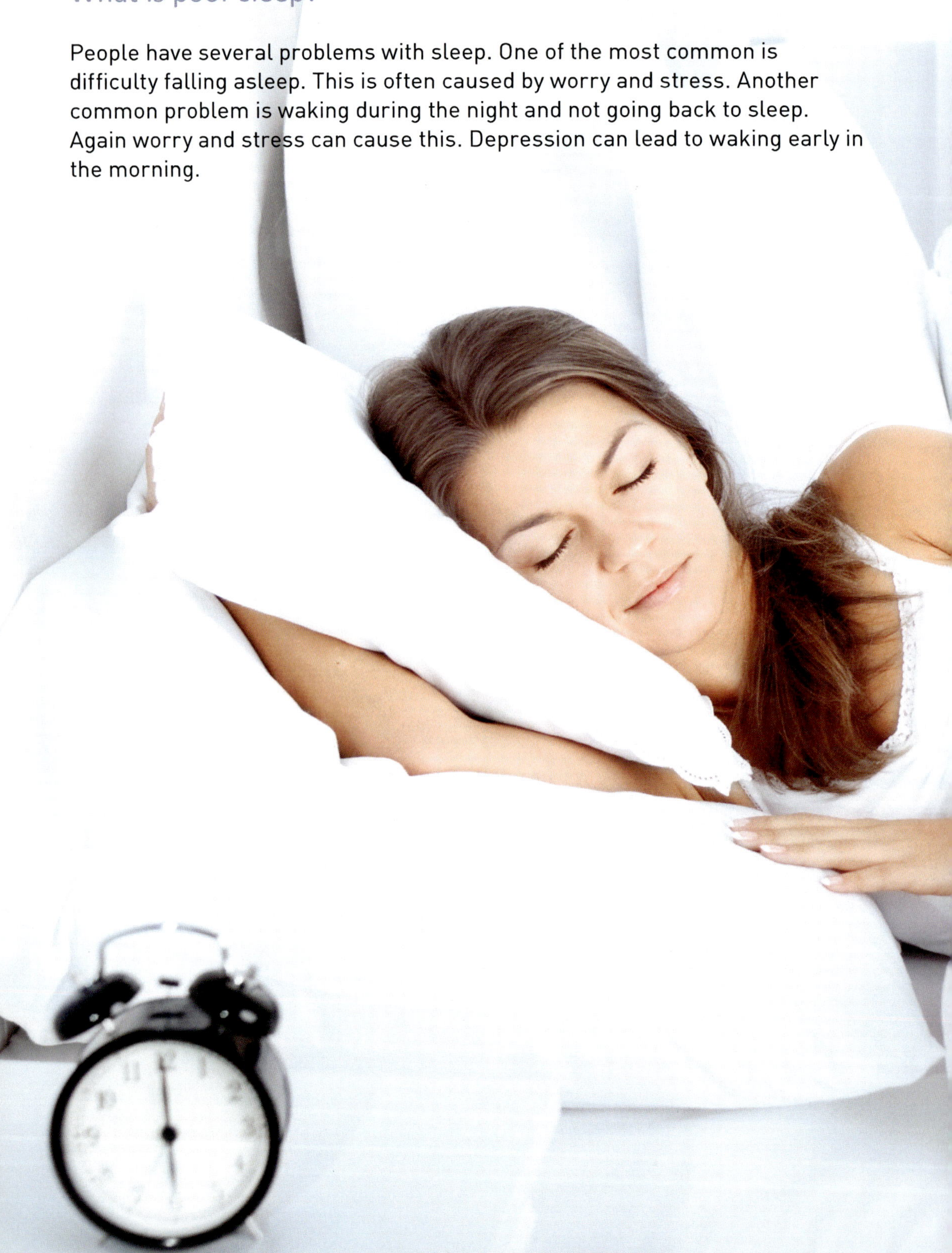

Sleep hygiene

TIP

A milky drink or protein meal in the evening gives you the essential amino acid, tryptophan, which aids sleep.

Try to keep your bedroom as dark as possible as even small amounts of light can disrupt your sleep hormones. Get good amounts of light during the day – at least an hour to stimulate good circadian rhythm, then have low light for an hour before you go to bed to allow good levels of melatonin. Try to avoid blue light at night, including blue clock lights. A red bulb or torch is a good way to read in bed to avoid blue light, especially if your partner likes a dark room. Keep the bedroom cool – about 20 degrees is the ideal.

Reserve the bedroom for sleeping. Turn off TVs and electrical appliances at the wall to reduce the electromagnetic field. If you must charge your phone or other device in the bedroom, move it as far as possible away from your bed.

Your bedtime routine should relax you. Essential oils, a good book or relaxing music help the body and mind to wind down ready for sleep.

Don't use the computer within an hour of bedtime and stop all work activities, too. Get into a habit or writing down all the jobs you have to do the next day, then draw a line under the list. Put it in your office or kitchen and then relax for the night so that you switch off from work well before you go to bed.

Reduce TV watching just before bed. Avoid stimulating drinks such as caffeine after 5pm or even lunchtime. Alcohol may help you to nod off but your liver metabolises the alcohol so it may make you wake up in the middle of the night. It also interferes with the quality of your sleep and prevents deep sleep when your body does most of its healing.

Try to establish a good routine – bedtime and getting up should be about the same time every day.

Try to have two to three nights a week with no alcohol so that you have good quality sleep with no interruptions.

Do exercise regularly during the day to help you relax.

Exercise overload and relaxation

Overtraining can lead to underperformance and chronic fatigue. It can also make you more susceptible to infection and illness.

Over-trainers may also experience more colds, headaches, muscle soreness, anxiety, mood imbalance and poor quality sleep.

When you overtrain results will plateau, you may experience more injuries, and often your energy levels become low. This is the result of your body telling you it's time for rest and recovery.

Habits that promote active recovery after exercise improve performance, strength and overall energy.

Active recovery

A rest day, and not necessarily a day of sitting on the couch!

Light exercise such as walking is low intensity and allows for the delivery of oxygen to the muscles. This increases blood flow to your muscles, hence better transportation of nutrients.

A great way to feel refreshed and rejuvenated!

Passive recovery

This is where, yes, you can sit on the couch! Usually saved for illness or injury.

TIPS

- Take regular holidays or weekend breaks.
- Say 'no' and keep your day free for you.
- Get adequate sleep.
- Smile!

Teenagers going vegetarian

This is a common issue and so many teenagers don't do it the right way. We applaud their ethical reasons for going vegetarian but they need to do it properly so they don't miss out on important nutrients. I've seen too many teenagers end up with depression and anxiety because they don't eat the right foods and a balanced vegetarian diet. Mostly they take a Western diet and just remove the meat. This is a recipe for disaster.

The first step in going vegetarian is to look at where you will get protein. Teenagers are still growing and often play sport so their requirements are quite high. Growth can be stunted by a low protein diet. Vegetarian sources of protein include nuts and seeds, soy, cheese and eggs as well as beans and legumes. Cheese and eggs, being animal products, are 25 per cent protein. So 100g of cheese will give 25g of protein. Vegetarian sources of protein contain less, so beans contain only 10per cent protein.

An average teenager weighing 70kg would need 70g-100g of protein a day. This would amount to 400g of cheese or egg, or 1kg of beans. So it's important to get enough protein and from a variety of sources. A good example for this teenager would be 100g cheese, 100g egg, 100g soy, 250g beans or legumes.

Vitamins and minerals are important. Iron, zinc and iodine are vital minerals. Iron can be obtained from molasses and greens such as spinach, zinc from nuts and seeds especially pepitas, and iodine from seaweed. Lack of iron causes tiredness and low zinc causes depression and anxiety and loss of appetite.

Most vitamins can be derived from vegetables. Vitamin B12 can be low if they don't eat dairy food. Vitamin D is obtained mostly from sunlight, so getting outside is important, too. Omega-3 is a marine oil, so if no fish is eaten then it's hard to get enough. Supplements in this case will help.

Unfortunately, many young vegetarians don't eat much vegetables. Chips and cola could be considered vegetarian. So as a parent your role is to make sure they are getting enough protein and the other necessary nutrients.

TIP

Have your child see a nutritionist to make sure they are 'eating from the rainbow' and getting as many nutrients as possible before supplements are needed.

Device and screen time

It's the bugbear of modern parenting. How to drag your little gem away from the computer screen or TV. Parents despair of sunny afternoons wasted indoors and with teenagers who won't leave their room.

This is a parental control issue. There is no point expecting the child to monitor their usage. They just don't have the wisdom and self-control. You have to take control of the situation and stick to good habits from the word go. When they're toddlers it's easy to give them your phone while you talk to the doctor or distract them with a funny game while you're driving. But make sure you set the boundaries, even at this age. Count the minutes your young child spends online or playing games. Online time should be seen as a privilege to be earned.

Create screen-free family time by picking two weekdays where there are no electronics. As well as this, set weekday and weekend time limits and adhere to them strictly. Kids are often grumpy and irritable after long sessions online, so be prepared to have to stick to your guns. Have a specific place in the loungeroom or familyroom where devices are placed each evening before bed.

Monitor your child's usage. Younger ones should use the internet in a family room so you can monitor the sites they access and who they're talking to. If there is bullying, sometimes you can intervene and stop it before it becomes a problem. I once got onto a bully by stating I was the mother and was going to print her messages and show them to her mother. The bullying stopped immediately. The same goes for phones. Check their phones for signs of bullying texts and social media. Talk to your children about bullying. Make sure they understand what it is and to talk to you about it. Use stories to illustrate when taunting and insults are not OK.

A camping holiday is great opportunity to break device habits, so make the rules clear early, that the family camping trip will be screen-free.

In the car it's tempting to put on a video or a game, so children come to expect that every trip will involve screentime. Make sure you have gadget-free trips, so that children have to talk and look out the window. Play games such as 'I spy' where they have to observe their surroundings.

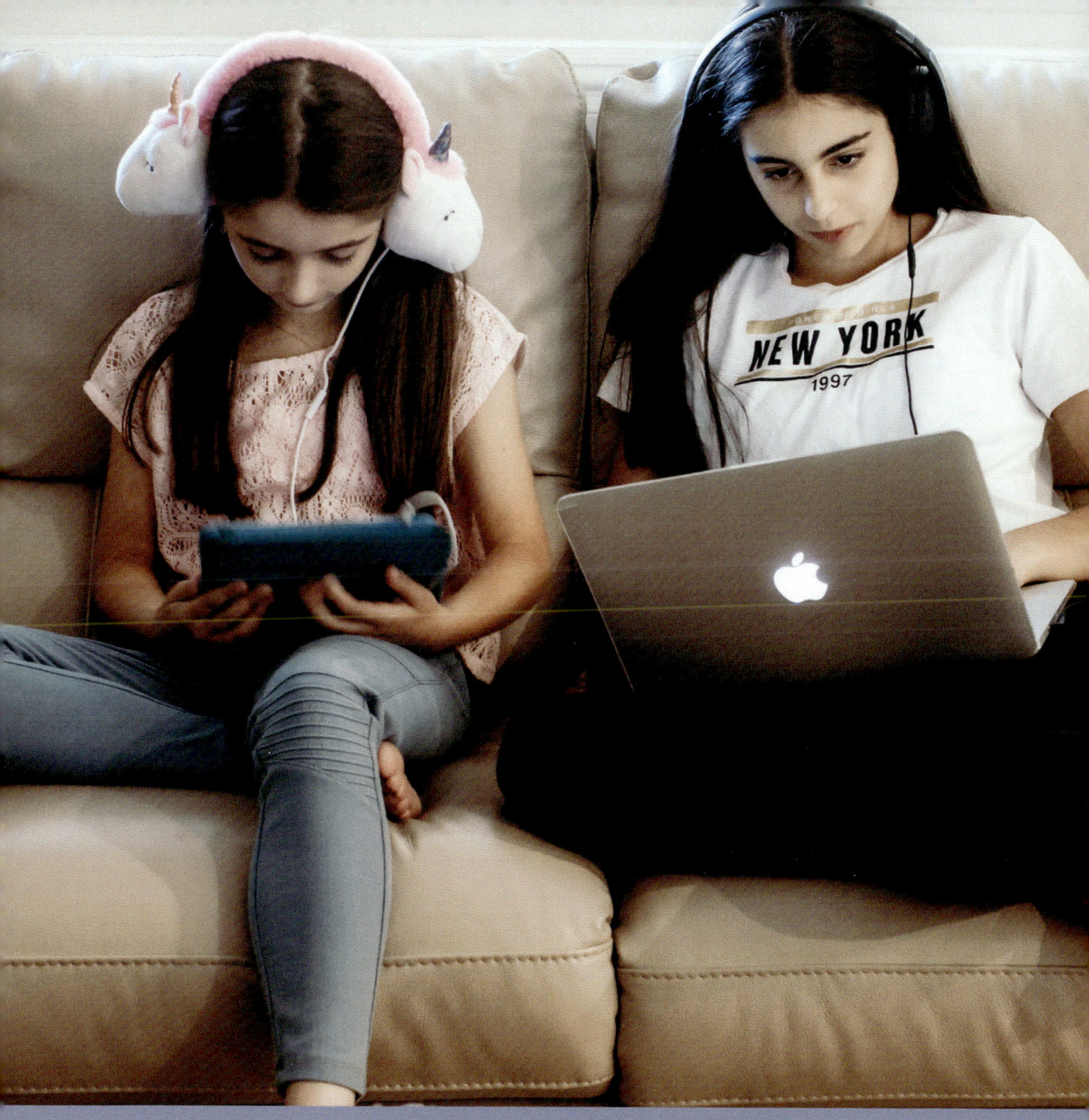

Buy a few audiobooks so the kids, and you, can listen to a story on the drive – you can discuss the story afterwards. Sing-along CDs or a Spotify playlist for carpool karaoke are also useful.

We lived in the Middle East when our kids were small and sometimes had 10-hour drives to a favourite campsite. Audiobooks were an amazing asset to pass the time with five people and a large dog squashed into the car.

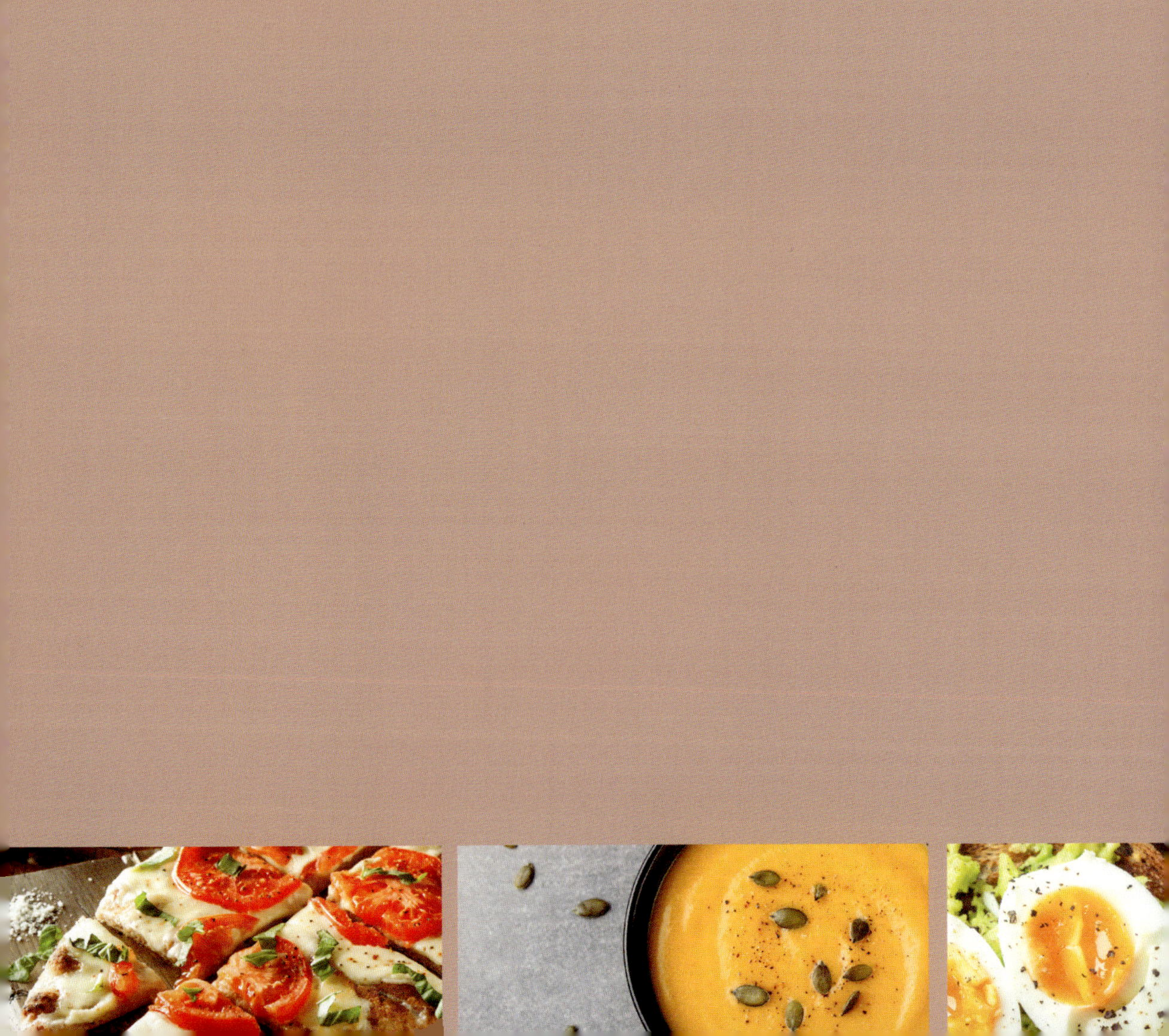

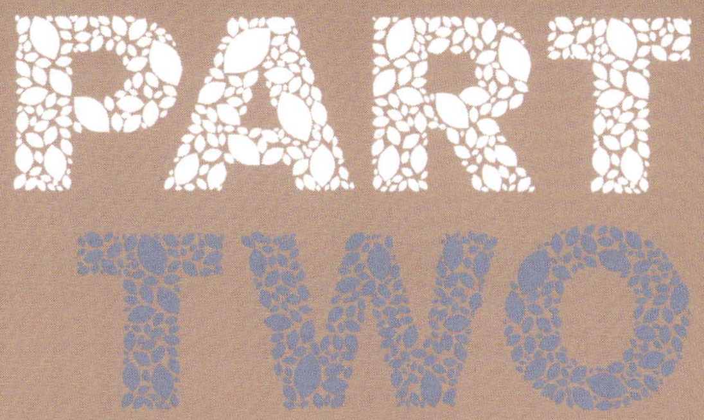

PART TWO

The specifics

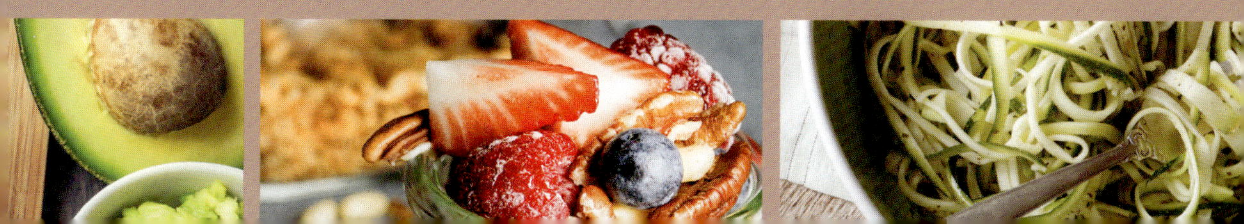

Allergies

Many children have allergies ranging from hay fever to peanuts. There are many theories about why it is such a problem but most experts agree that good gut health goes a long way to help reduce the number of allergies a child has.

The gut biome has millions of bacteria that originally come from our surroundings. Breastfeeding and also baby probiotics help establish a good microbiome. Letting your child get dirty and play out in the garden or in a sandpit is a great way to expose them to healthy bacteria to colonise the gut. It also helps keep the immune system busy so it doesn't overreact to foods.

I'm not a fan of anti-bacterial handwash. Our hands are already covered in healthy bacteria and that's normal. We don't want to wash those healthy bacteria away! I would just use regular soap for daily use and anti-bacterial handwash only if someone has a cold.

Ideally, you want your child to develop a healthy immune system that reacts to infections but does not overreact to foods, so giving them a healthy diet can feed the immune system with the nutrients it needs to perform properly. A healthy diet means avoiding processed foods that contain additives and colourings, because they can excite the brain and cause behavioural problems.

If your child does develop a food allergy, seek expert help. There are many options to solve the problem, from symptom relievers to desensitisation drops. Don't restrict your child's diet too much as they may end up lacking important nutrients. Get help before you reach the stage of a very limited diet. Rather than restricting foods, fixing the gut biome goes a long way to managing allergies.

Anxiety

Anxiety is becoming more common at all ages. Children in particular can become anxious about family breakups, bullying at school, and even the news. There are many things you can do to help reduce anxiety in your child, whether it's fear of the dark or of flying.

First of all, a healthy diet is important. The brain works with various hormones and neurotransmitters and the building blocks of these hormones are vitamins and minerals. Make sure they get a balanced diet of healthy protein, veggies, and fruit. Ditch the processed stuff, especially in the lunch box.

Omega-3 is also vitally important. Our brain cells are covered in a fatty layer, the myelin sheath. When we're short of Omega-3, that covering is thin and patchy, making the nerves irritable – just like an exposed electrical wire without its plastic covering. This can make us irritable and anxious. So get some kids' fish oil and make sure they take it regularly. If you are vegetarian, then Udo's oil with DHA is a good plant source of Omega-3. It tastes like sesame, so I mix it with hommus to disguise the taste.

We all know parenting is hard and there is no rule book. But one of the most important parts of parenting is spending time with your children and being available to listen to them. In our busy world, it's too easy to use the electronic babysitters of TV and computer games, so that while they're quiet, you can get on with chores. Parents it is an absolute must to spend some time each day chatting to your child and listening to them. Family time around the dinner table is a great way to have an informal chat and a good habit to get into. Or have some family downtime together where there's no TV or other distraction.

Encourage your child to talk about their worries and comfort them when they are upset. It's very important to set up these habits so that when they become teenagers they are used to coming to you for help, knowing you'll listen. That way, you'll be in the loop about what they're doing and who they're hanging out with.

Build confidence in your children so that they're happier in themselves. If they can't catch a ball well, spend a few Saturdays practising with them. Pick something they think they are no good at and show them that a bit of practice can go a long way. Many kids believe talent is something you're born with. They don't understand that practice and training are the key to success. Many elite athletes started with no visible talent but devoted themselves to becoming great. The more skills your child can pick up, the more confident they will be.

I see so many kids who are exhausted from being run all over town every afternoon, so don't overdo the after-school activities. Make sure they have at least two school days where they just come home and relax. When my son was six, I couldn't find him to take him to tennis lessons. He was hiding under the bed and said 'I'm tired, I just want to stay home and play with my toys'. After that I was more careful about not pushing him too hard. Kids who are introverts may find school exhausting and need some time on their own to unwind, so have some space in their room to de-stress in peace and quiet before hitting the homework.

Finally, try to be a good role model for your children. Many young people see drama on TV in which everyone freaks out over every little incident. They think this is real life and that freaking out is the appropriate response. Freaking out never achieves anything and is a waste of energy. We all have to face problems every day, but luckily most of us never have to face the daily problems of starvation, lack of water, and the threat of violence that many countries in the developing world endure daily.

So, put your problems into perspective. Your son might not get into the school you wanted. That's annoying, but in the scheme of things it's not a massive problem. Having a minor accident in your car is frustrating, but be glad nobody died. Most of our problems are minor and need only a bit of problem-solving. There is most likely a solution to the problems you are facing and you just need time to think about them. So keep calm, model good problem-solving behaviour and your kids will follow your lead.

If you can't see a way through, or it's a larger problem, seek help from a professional. You don't need to deal with those big problems alone.

Body image

Social media has been a great help to many businesses and getting health information out to people. But the massive downside is one we could not have predicted. Body shaming and Instagram bloggers with perfect bodies have distorted our view of what is normal.

People come in all shapes and sizes and we often can't change that. Maybe in the future, we'll all live in virtual bodies and look like Lara Croft, but until that day we have to accept that some people will be short and some will be stocky and not everyone will have a long-legged willowy body fit for a model.

Unfortunately, we are bombarded with pictures of perfect bodies that make us feel inadequate. It's difficult enough for adults to deal with the feelings we have when we look at these toned yoga bodies, but it's even worse for children.

When we look in the mirror, we tend to exaggerate our imperfections and feel we look bigger or smaller than we are. Eventually we become distressed or ashamed every time we look in the mirror. This is called body dysmorphia.

Danger signals in your child include:

1. Refusing to look in the mirror or undress in front of others
2. Refusal to wear a swimsuit or go swimming
3. Depression or withdrawal from socialising
4. Self-harm such as picking at skin or eyelashes
5. Extreme starvation, diets, or bingeing, followed by vomiting.

Our girls and boys and young women and men need to be directed away from judging themselves purely on how they look.

There are many smart and successful women and it's our job to encourage our girls and young women to find their strengths and where they can do good in the world. Why should women feel the need to have a perfect body to be womanly? These are old values that we need to smash.

Encourage your girls to value themselves for reasons other than their looks. They might be smart or extrovert or caring or good at sports. Think widely about the attributes they have that are worth celebrating. Remind them constantly how good their skills are and boost their confidence.

Teach them good communication, introduce them to other adults, and role play meeting strangers, for example, at work, or teachers and tutors. Girls tend to be better at this than boys but some shy or introvert girls and boys need help learning to talk to people. These will be great skills to have when they start to look for work.

Public speaking is one of our biggest fears, but it's an invaluable skill. Most people will have to make some sort of presentation in their working life, so have your children practise giving speeches in your safe, home environment. The only effective way to conquer fear of public speaking is to do it over and over, until there is no fear left. Often girls like to put on plays – so encourage this. Get them to recite poetry or sing songs, and get the boys involved too. After some time, introduce other adults to the audience so they get used to performing in front of strangers.

Finally, be a good role model. If you're off getting botoxed every week and buying lots of clothes, this will reinforce the message that looks are more important than anything else.

We often think body dysmorphia is focused on girls, but boys have body image issues too. Depending on their age, this may be thinking they are over weight, wanting to be thinner, or more muscular. Keeping them active, enjoying the outdoors, eating healthily, and staying away from computer games, will help them build skills that boost their confidence and help develop an outward-looking attitude.

Encourage your children to recycle old clothes and accessories and reinforce environmentally sound shopping. Make saving the world, making a difference, and contributing to the community more important than having a perfect body and you'll have made a great start on building confident, worldly wise children.

Chronic fatigue

While not common in children, it can be a real problem to diagnose. Chronic fatigue can have many causes so it's best to consult an expert if you're worried. Teenagers often appear fatigued, especially during growth spurts.

Many children do not get enough sleep and so are constantly in sleep debt. If they are often tired, try getting them into a new sleep pattern by going to bed early for two weeks so they get at least eight hours' sleep. Reduce sport or other commitments and increase fluids to make sure they are getting at least two litres of water a day.

If your child is still tired, consult a doctor and have some simple blood tests. Iron deficiency is common. Low levels of zinc and B12 can be the first sign of gut problems. Unfortunately, the reference ranges for many of these tests, that is, the value deemed normal for a healthy person, are too low. The results are compared with those of people who are sick and often elderly and do not reflect the range for optimal health, especially in young people. Children who are growing and playing lots of sport burn through lots of vitamins and minerals every day.

Child athletes are becoming more common with gymnasts, runners and swimmers starting at younger ages. Overtraining and exhaustion are common and burnout is the result. I have seen many children who are fed up with their sport but are not allowed to give it up because of their ambitious parents. Rest days are *so* important and at least two rest days a week are needed for muscles to grow, repair, and recover. If your child wants to stop the sport, let them have a rest for a term. Sometimes time off is all that's required to rekindle their interest.

If none of the above is working, it's time to consider more serious causes. Unfortunately, we don't have any good tests for fatigue, so it's all about the symptoms. If your child is short of breath during exercise when they weren't before, have lost fitness, or take a long time to recover, it's time to think of other causes, so consult your doctor.

Do they have Epstein Barr virus or other infections such as Ross River fever? Your doctor should be able to test for these. Lyme disease, an infection caused by the tick-borne bacteria Borrelia is now seen in Australia. And lastly, contact with mould. Mould illness is now recognised as a big problem worldwide and a common cause of fatigue. Children may be affected by mould in their bedroom, mattress, or bathroom. Also think about other contact with mould such as at school, work, or sports and hobby venues. Damp and underused scout halls are common places where mould grows.

If you suspect any of these issues, consult an expert in chronic fatigue to get the right testing done. The good news is that all of these can be treated and often get great results.

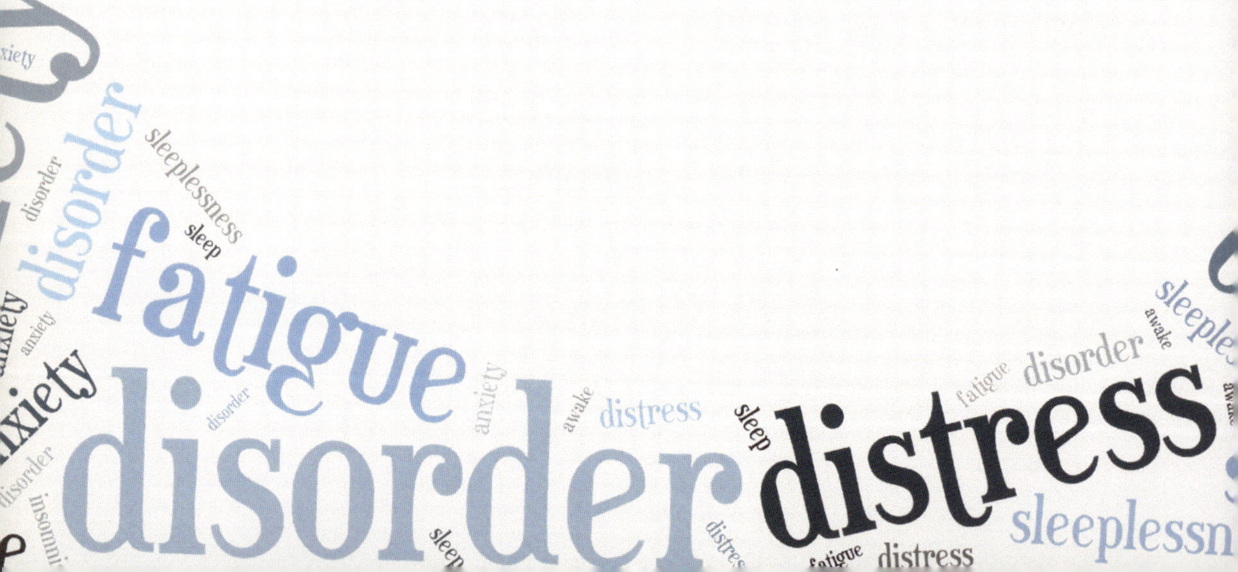

Coeliac and gluten sensitivity

True coeliac disease is not as common as you'd think but many people are gluten intolerant. Unfortunately, testing is rarely helpful. Blood tests such as TTG antibodies (tissue transglutaminase) are rarely positive unless the child is eating a high gluten diet. The gene test for coeliac, HLD–DQ2 and HLA-DQ8 genes, indicate a likelihood of coeliac disease.

The only reliable test for coeliac disease is a gastroscopy, a camera is sent down into the stomach and small intestine to have a look. I find an elimination diet for a month and then a challenge of lots of bread for three days helps people tell if wheat gluten is a problem for them.

Gluten intolerance occurs when there is no coeliac disease but the patient still has problems with gluten, such as pain, bloating, gas and diarrhoea or constipation. Gluten can also cause leaky gut. The only solution is to go gluten free. Sometimes with gluten intolerance, after six months people can tolerate a small amount of gluten such as birthday cake, but it's best not to eat gluten every day.

Gluten is present in many foods, especially cereal grains, but it is mostly the gluten in wheat and oats that is a problem. Many people can safely eat rice, gluten-free products, barley, corn, and quinoa. Buckwheat and chia are not cereal grains and are usually fine.

So it's best to remove all bread and pastries, muffins, pasta, white, or flour sauces. Sweets, ice-cream and any processed food often have hidden wheat. Safe foods include white rice, potato, sweet potato, pumpkin, meat, fish, fruit, and vegetables.

It can be difficult if the rest of the family continues to eat bread, when the child with gluten intolerance cannot. It also takes time to understand all the sources of wheat gluten and how to avoid them. Luckily, there are many websites and coeliac societies to help you remove gluten from your child's diet.

Constipation

Constipation in children, adolescents, and even adults is rather common. There is usually no major cause and a change in diet and an increase in fluid intake will usually fix the issue. But what is normal when it comes to frequency of bowel movements? Ideally you should be going to the bathroom daily. There should be no pain and no other symptoms such as a sore belly or loss of appetite.

If we examine the things we should be doing to avoid constipation we need to look closely at our diet, particularly our fibre and fluid intake.

Most of us don't get enough fibre because our vegetable intake is minimal. Fluid needs to be just water, not packaged milk drinks, soft drink, or caffeinated energy drinks. Drinking enough water helps stools move more easily through the intestines but the amount kids, teens, and adults need will vary based on their activity, weight, and age.

Some causes of constipation

- Diet too low in fibre
- Gluten intolerance
- Water intake is low
- Diet is high in processed foods
- Too many fatty or spicy foods
- Drinking too much cow's milk
- Certain medications
- Stress and anxiety
- Irritable bowel syndrome.

To do list

- Increase water by 500ml a day
- Try not to eat the same thing every day, have more variety
- Try some prunes or prune juice, warm apple or pear
- Include fresh fruit and vegetables daily, particularly greens
- Exercise more
- See your doctor if you have abdominal pain, pain when passing your stools, or if you have not been to the toilet for five days.

Diabetes/insulin resistance

Normally when you eat sugar, your pancreas makes insulin, which helps you move sugar out of the blood stream and into your cells for energy. If you eat too much sugar, your pancreas has to work very hard to make a lot of insulin.

Diabetes has two distinct types. Type 2 diabetes happens when a person who has genes for diabetes, eats too much sugar and carbohydrates over a long period. The pancreas eventually gets tired and can't make enough insulin. At the same time, the insulin that is made does not get the message through and this is called insulin resistance. Finally, the patient needs tablets or even injections of insulin to control the blood sugar.

Type 1 diabetes is totally different. This happens suddenly and usually in childhood. The pancreas is hit by a virus or similar problem and is no longer able to make insulin. From then on, the patient needs injections of insulin because the pancreas never recovers. Luckily, we have insulin pumps now that make life a lot easier without the need for daily injections. Stress is a big feature in Type 1 diabetes and can be provoked by childhood trauma such as divorce, family separation etc.

Historically, Type 2 diabetes occured in mainly older people because their diet was too high in sugar and carbs and they didn't exercise enough. Today we are seeing an increase in Type 2 diabetes in young people.

To prevent this, we need to reduce the amount of sugar children eat and encourage them to exercise. This trains the body to burn fat for energy rather than carbs and sugar. Adding healthy fats to the diet improves this problem, too. Olive oil added to salads and veggies, organic butter on potatoes, and coconut oil for stir frys, can be a great way to add healthy oils to your child's diet.

It's rare to find small children who are overweight because they run around so much. But a diet high in processed food, sugar and high carbs will encourage obesity as the child grows. So removing processed food is important, too.

Gut health and probiotics

This is a very important topic. We now realise that the gut affects many systems all over the body. Whenever someone has a disease, whether it's a mental or physical illness, the gut plays a part in the disease process and also the treatment. It's important to have plenty of good bacteria in the gut to produce healthy hormones but it's also important to have a healthy gut lining.

The gut lining acts as a barrier and prevents harmful chemicals and bacteria entering the body. If it breaks down, we get 'leaky gut'. This is quite common and means toxins and chemicals leech into the body causing pain and stiffness such as in our joints and muscles. A leaky gut is also not good at absorbing nutrients from our food.

So it's important to ensure your children have a healthy gut.

1. Regular probiotics: probiotics don't hang around long in the gut. But when there, they police the gut bacteria and keep them under control. They are important at the edge of the gut lining where healthy bacteria keep the gut barrier working well.

2. Prebiotics: these are important fuel for the gut and feed the healthy gut bacteria. Prebiotics occur in fresh vegetables, legumes and some grains.

3. Fermented foods also contain healthy probiotics and prebiotics. Try giving your child kombucha to drink from time to time. They may also like sauerkraut or kimchi. Fresh fermented yoghurt such as kefir is easy to make. Many supermarket brands of yoghurt have little healthy bacteria and have added sugar and artificial sweeteners. So try to buy plain biodynamically active yoghurt and add your own fruit.

4. Reduce processed food as it has chemicals such as emulsifiers that can break down the gut lining barrier.

5. Reduce sugar as it provides food for unhealthy bacteria such as candida.

A good gut will set your kids up for a healthy life.

Hormonal changes and hunger in adolescents

The teenage years are a time of raging hormones and severe mood swings. Girls are getting their periods earlier and earlier so are exposed to higher levels of oestrogen and progesterone at a younger age. Oestrogen stimulates metabolism and may decrease appetite. An imbalance of hormones may promote appetite and weight gain. A low thyroid is rare in children but older teenagers can suffer from a sluggish thyroid. This is usually due to not getting all the vitamins and minerals needed for good thyroid function.

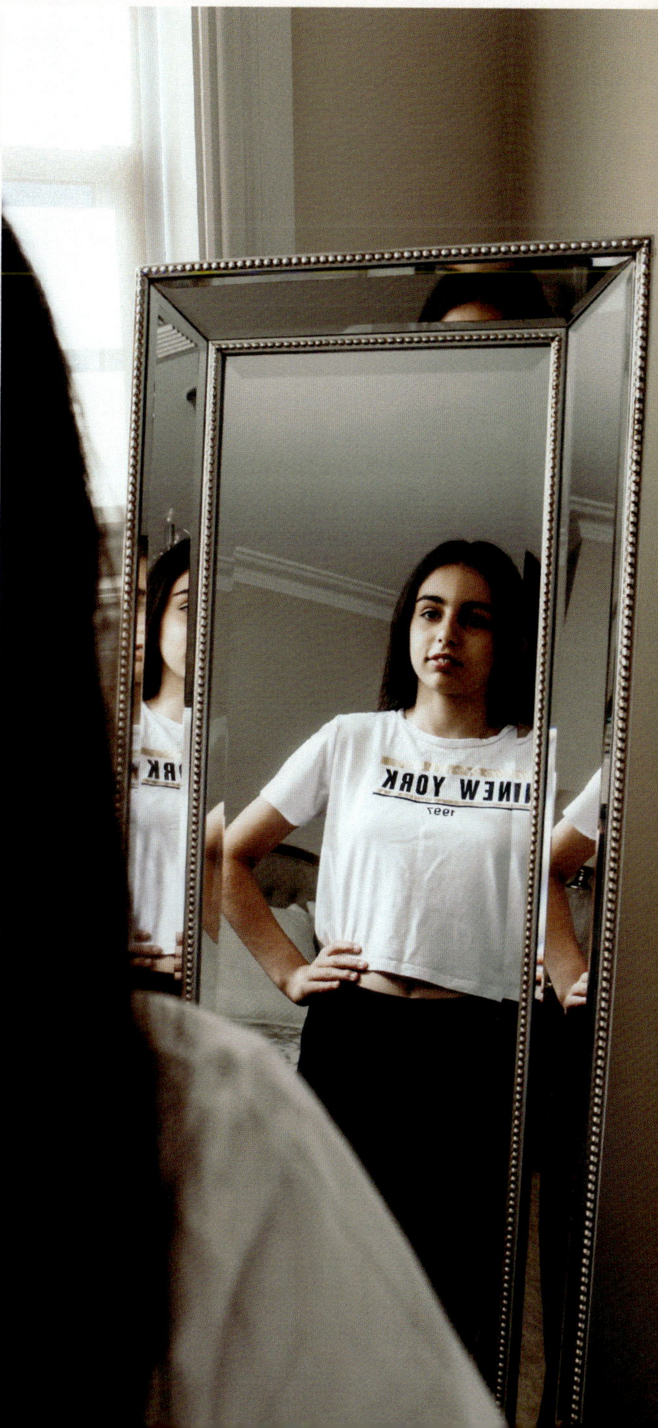

For boys, their requirements to make hormones such as testosterone during adolescence is huge. Zinc deficiency can become a problem as large amounts of zinc are needed to make testosterone. Low zinc can also stunt growth and cause boys to be irritable. Testing their levels and supplementing until levels return to normal can be important to stimulate growth and improve mood. Low blood sugar is also a common cause of being grumpy. Less sugar in the diet and more healthy oils helps to balance blood sugar and prevent low blood sugar.

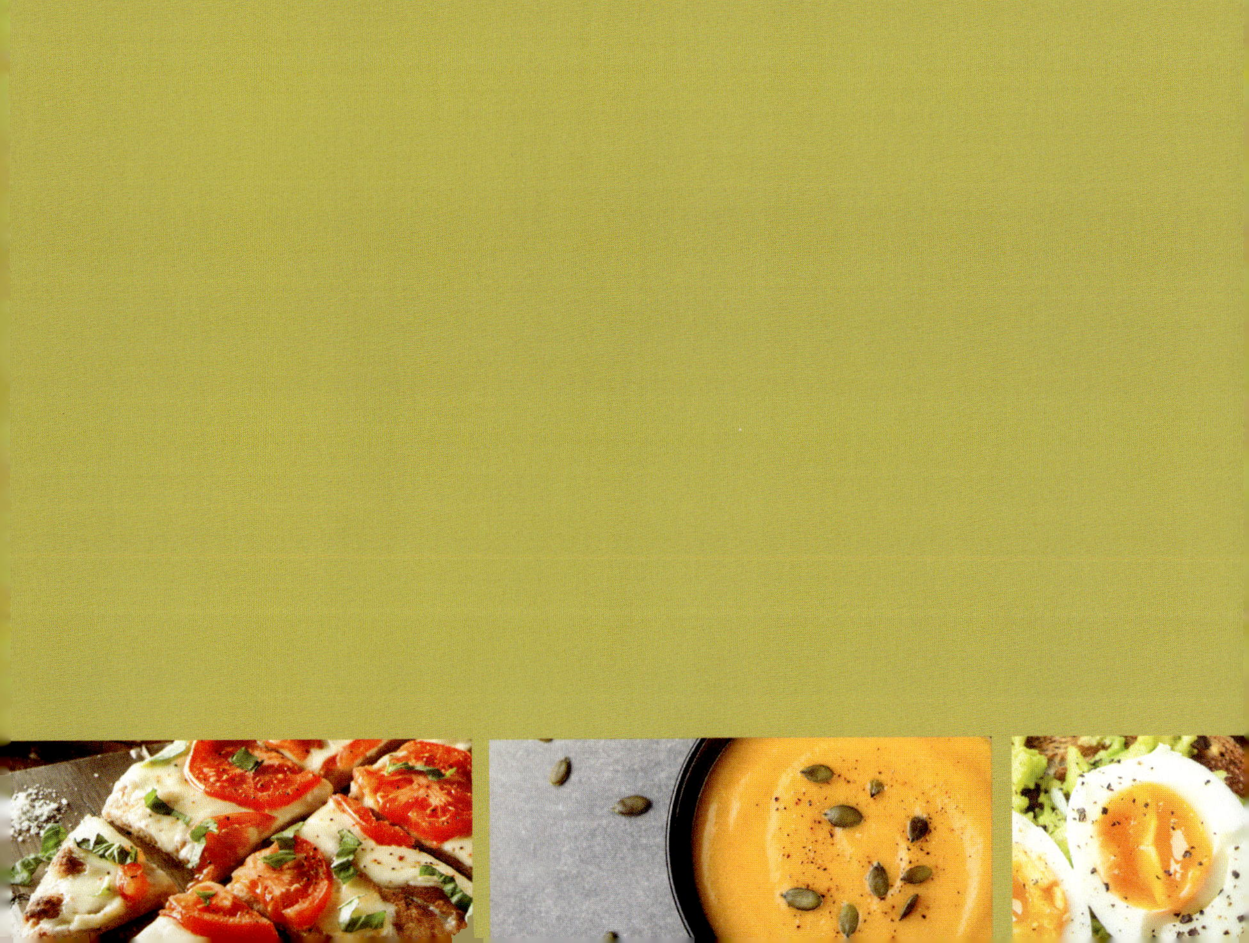

PART THREE

Back to school, after school, and party planning

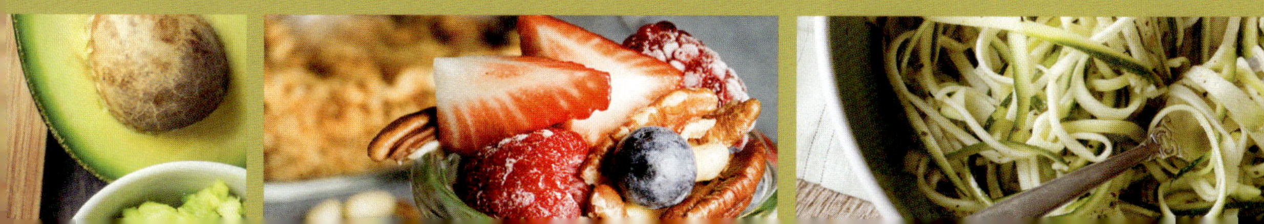

Back to school

That time of year when parents have a smile from ear to ear and school shoes, uniforms, and lunch boxes are on the to-do list!

Packing a healthy lunch does not require a fancy lunch box. It's all in the content. Remember, kids spend many hours at school so what they eat and how much they eat is important.

The snacks will depend on what's available and what is an approved snack.

See our App for approved supermarket items including snacks.

If you prefer to make your child's entire lunch box, that's OK too. Our philosophy at Foodfix is to let kids be kids. Not allowing them an ice block on a hot day occasionally is taking healthy eating to the extreme. We suggest to balance a treat with the rest of the lunch box and eating for that day.

Step 1: Lunch

You might make a sandwich, wrap, or roll. Try to include some protein and salad, for example, ham, avocado and lettuce, or chicken, avocado and lettuce.

If you have a fussy eater, a cheese and/or Vegemite sandwich is OK from time to time. Remember repetition gets boring, so the need for variety is important. For example try a wrap or roll instead of sliced bread every day. Change the fillings to include boiled eggs, left-over barbecue chicken, or vegetable patty.

Lunch can also be a cooked item such as egg muffin or frittata bites. Rice paper rolls also make a great lunch and snack. Just start with a protein and your child's favourite fillings.

Variety means not every day needs bread. You could also do a rice/pasta salad, or an open lunch of cut protein such as leftover chicken, cheese cubes, baby tomatoes, olives and a few crackers.

TIP

To keep lunch boxes fresh and cool, include a freezable ice brick.

Step 2: Fruit

Always include one small serving of fruit.

Step 3: Fluid

Always pack water! No juices or pre-packaged milk drinks are necessary. Not only are they highly processed but also contain unnecessary amounts of sugar.

Step 4: Snacks

Here we recommend one packaged item and one non-packaged item.

Approved packaged snacks include:

- Low-sugar muesli bar (See our App for approved varieties)
- Popcorn
- Cheese and biscuit snack packs
- Fava beans or chickpeas
- VitaWeats or rice cakes with Vegemite/peanut butter

Note: Always check your school's nut policy.

Non-packaged snacks include:

- Carrot and cucumber sticks with hommus/avocado dip
- Egg muffin, home-made low-sugar muffin, or frittata slice. See recipes on page 74
- Homemade seeded crackers
- Home-made, nut-free bliss balls. See recipe page 96, 99

Allowing your child to choose their snack just once a week will mean you're in the good books and really, only one treat has been given!

I do not like to pack yoghurt. I leave this as a refreshing after-school snack as it will be cold and you can add fresh fruit, nuts or muesli to keep your child satisfied until dinner.

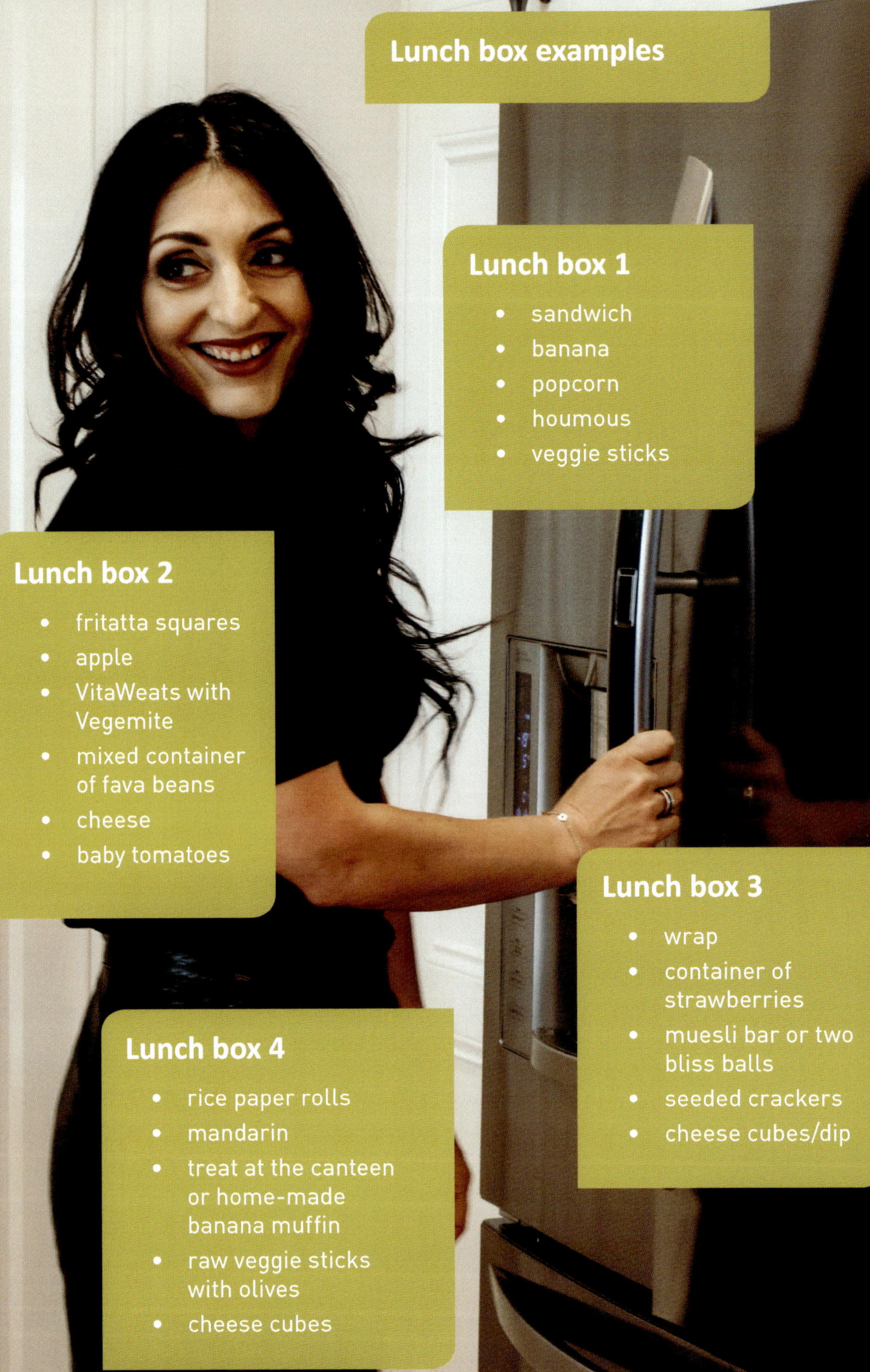

Lunch box examples

Lunch box 1

- sandwich
- banana
- popcorn
- houmous
- veggie sticks

Lunch box 2

- fritatta squares
- apple
- VitaWeats with Vegemite
- mixed container of fava beans
- cheese
- baby tomatoes

Lunch box 3

- wrap
- container of strawberries
- muesli bar or two bliss balls
- seeded crackers
- cheese cubes/dip

Lunch box 4

- rice paper rolls
- mandarin
- treat at the canteen or home-made banana muffin
- raw veggie sticks with olives
- cheese cubes

After school

They will be hungry. Perhaps starving. This is normal and usually means either:

- They are not getting enough fuel during the day
- They may not be drinking enough water.

If this is the case try an extra snack in the lunch box or a hearty high protein afternoon tea snack. When kids are super hungry, they will grab whatever is easier (usually processed rubbish) so make sure you have cut veggies/other good snacks on hand. Our after school snack suggestions are:

Yoghurt for when they come home. This means they will have a fresh, cold snack to which you can add a few tablespoons of muesli or some nuts and seeds, if they are really hungry.

VitaWeats or rice cakes with peanut butter are crunchy when fresh. Try adding some banana and a dash of cinnamon for a great tasting snack.

Rice paper rolls are fun to make and kids can generally put together their own with simple fillings such as ham and cucumber. These are also great for before sport.

Egg muffins have always been a winner in our house. They are filling and high in protein with a serve of vegetables. They are perfect to grab-and-go and great for a quick snack before after-school activities. Try making these on the weekend to get the kids involved and use their favourite ingredients such as bacon, ham, mushroom, and cheese. See recipe on page 74.

Bliss Balls are another great recipe for the kids to manage either on their own or with your help. These are great to grab-and-go, as a quick snack after sport, or even as a treat after dinner. Note: as they contain nuts these are not for school. See our recipes for nut-free versions on page 96, 99.

Tip-You can use the chocolate bliss ball as a base and add peppermint, orange, coffee (for the older kids and parents) to your child's liking. Don't make them too big. About 35-40g is a serve size. These keep in the freezer for ages. Just take them out and let them sit for 10 minutes before you take a bite. See recipe on page 96.

Party planning the healthy way

When planning a great party, sugar can become a parent's worst nightmare. You know a party means fun but it also means copious amounts of party food. So take the less is more approach. Plan your menu with your child, make a list and execute. As kids become teenagers, the party menu changes, and attire, location, and music become the focus.

There is always cake, so how do we make this healthier? I like to have one small cake to cut with friends then offer cupcakes for the guests/kids. These are usually smaller than an average slice of cake so contain less sugar. If funding doesn't allow this, cut a larger cake into coffee serves. Offering guests cake to take home instead of eating at the party is another way to encourage them to eat some of the other, healthier, food on offer.

Next would be a tray of various sandwiches, wraps, and rolls. These are simple to make and will also satisfy any adults at the party. Always offer the basics such as cheese and Vegemite and you will be surprised how quickly they are eaten. Be creative here and also have a selection of bread types to make the platter look more appealing.

Then comes fruit. Depending on the age of the children I have done fruit on a stick for the juniors and fruit cups or a platter for the older ones. On a hot day fruit is refreshing and tends to be a winner with the adults too.

My last platter is always cheese, veggie sticks, and a dip. I stick to one dip such as avocado or hommus, lots of crackers including the low carb ones, and just two varieties of cheese. I usually cut cheese pieces or cubes because they are easy to pick up and eat with a cracker.

Try putting the dip in small single-serve container pots with a carrot or cucumber sticking out of it. This eliminates double dipping.

For teenagers, planning the menu together is important. Having your child's input is the way to go. Platters are usually similar, but on a smaller scale with some raw treats if there are no nut allergies.

So where are the lollies and chips you ask? You can put single serve packs in a lolly bag for your guests to take home and consume in moderation.

What about hot food? It's generally not necessary, but pizza is a popular request from teenagers. They like to keep it simple to have more talk time. Try to make them yourself, if you have the time. If ordering in, go for thin-crust, wood-fired pizzas with less cheese/processed meat.

Healthy food menu

Menu suggestion: Kids

- Assorted sandwiches, wraps, or mini bread rolls
- Fruit sticks, cups, fruit platter, or ice pops in summer. See recipe pages.
- Platter of cheese, veggie sticks, and a selection of nut-free bliss balls
- The cake.

Menu suggestion: Teenagers

- Platter of assorted sandwiches and mini rolls
- Pizza, home-made nachos with avocado dip and natural corn chips, crackers or even rice paper rolls. See recipe pages.
- Cheese, crackers, nuts, bliss balls, and a fruit platter
- Cake, raw treats, or banana bites. See recipe pages.

Tips

- Get creative with the healthy stuff
- Limit the sweets
- Less is more
- Water only, no soft drinks
- Party time should be two to three hours maximum
- Check for allergies, gluten or other intolerances.

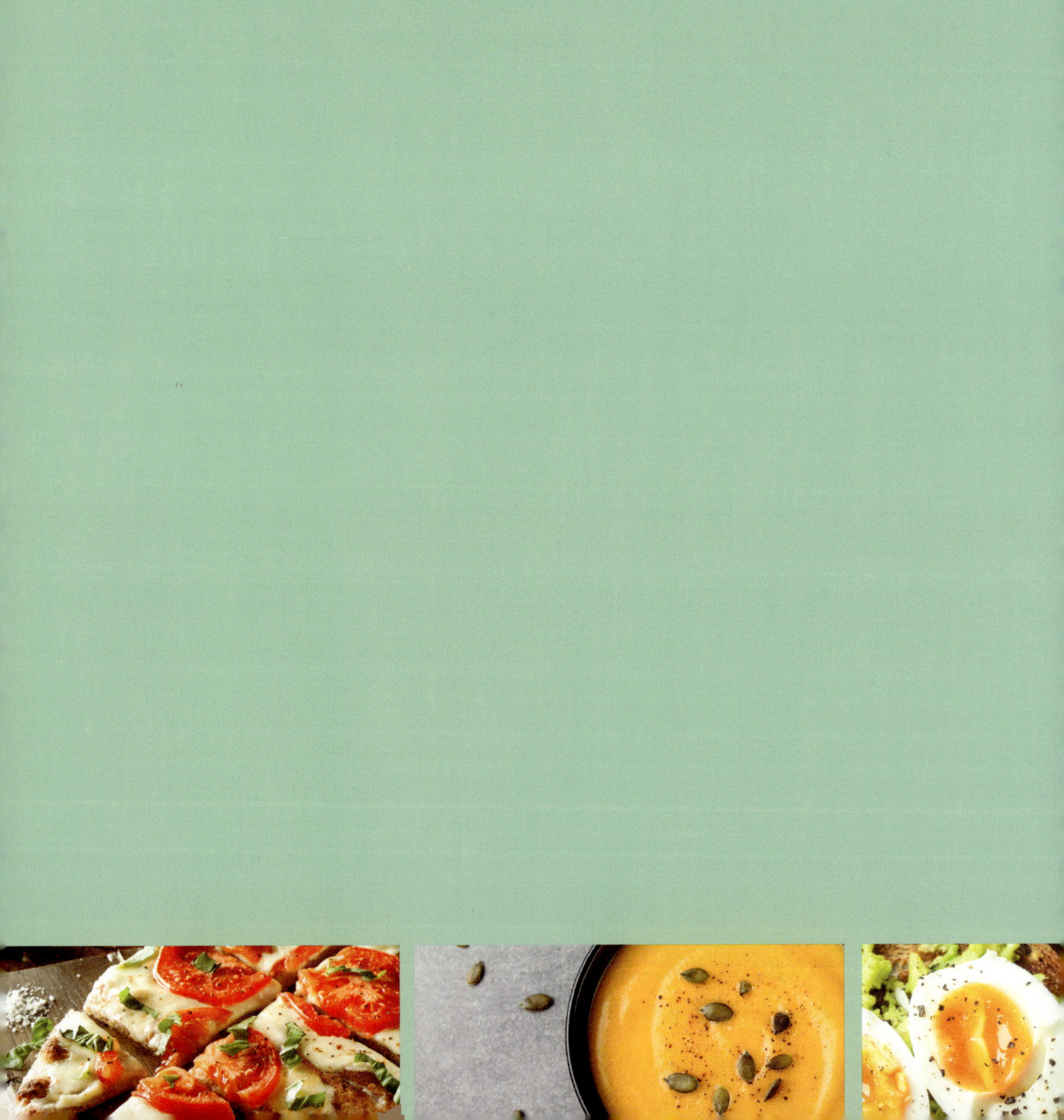

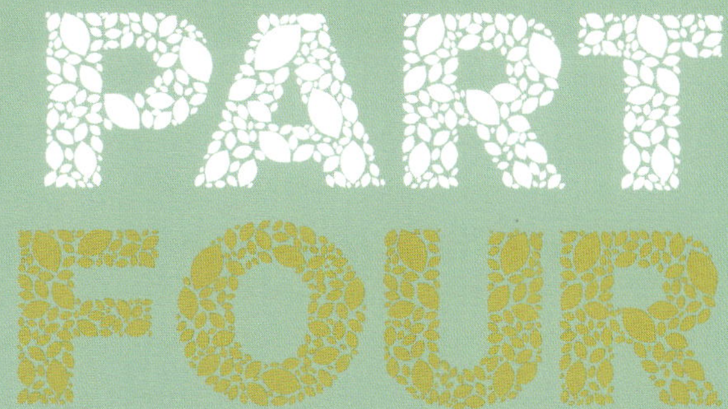

Recipes

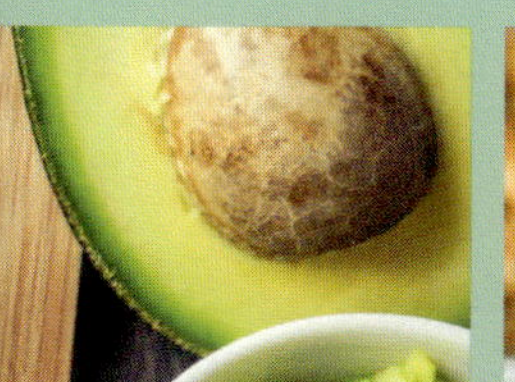

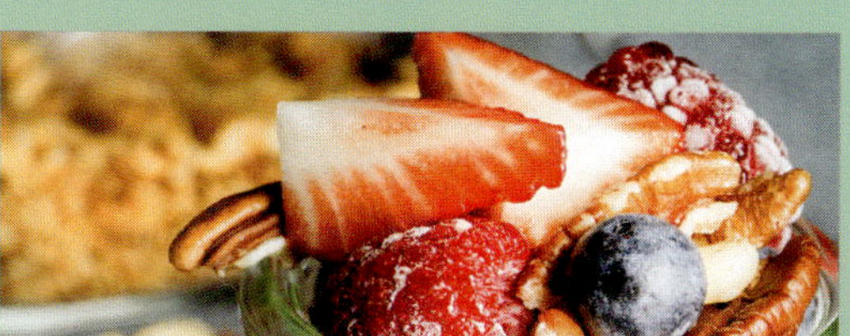

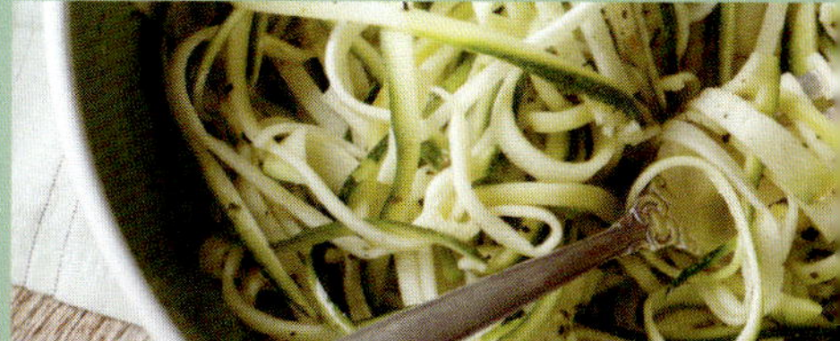

Breakfast 52

On the Go Snacks 74

Lunch & Dinner 110

Dessert 148

Omelette with spinach

SERVES
1

This makes a great breakfast, lunch or dinner. You can add your favourite veggies, additional protein and some cheese for a tasty, hearty meal.

Ingredients

3 eggs *or* 4 egg whites

Handful spinach

Handful mushrooms or other veggies you have on hand

Method

1. Whisk eggs and pour into heated pan sprayed with extra virgin olive oil spray to prevent sticking.
2. Add spinach and mushrooms and allow to cook for a few minutes
3. With a spatula fold over once and cook for a few more minutes.

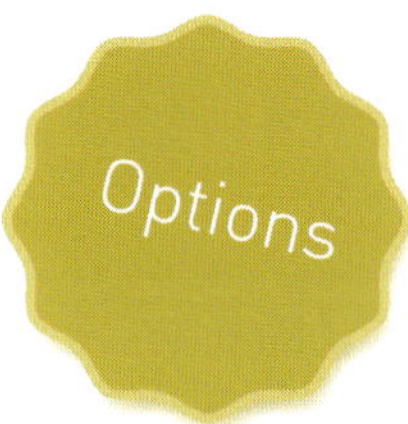

Try the following combinations:

Fetta cheese, smoked salmon and onion

Ham, cheese and tomato

Spinach, mushroom, red capsicum and fetta

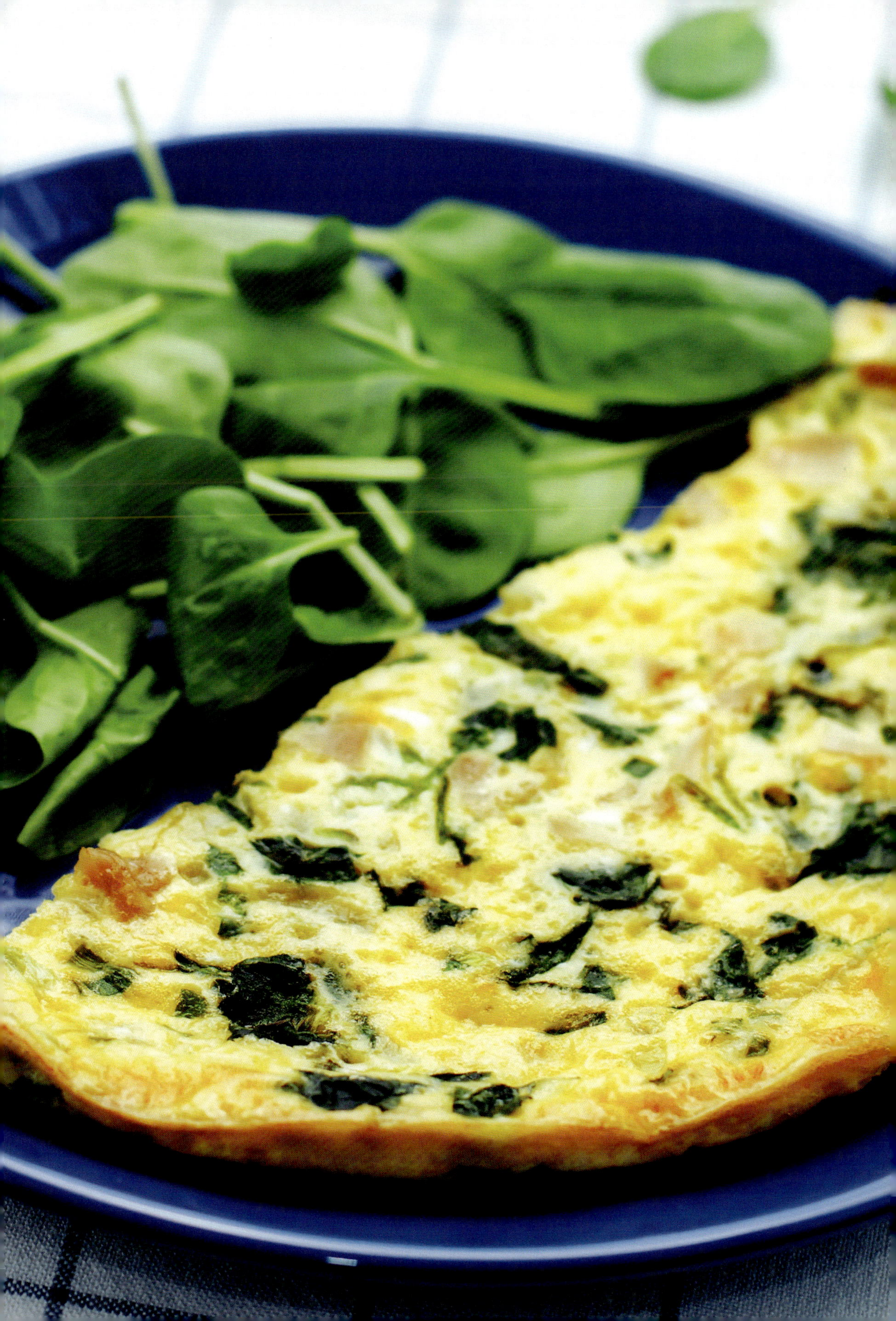

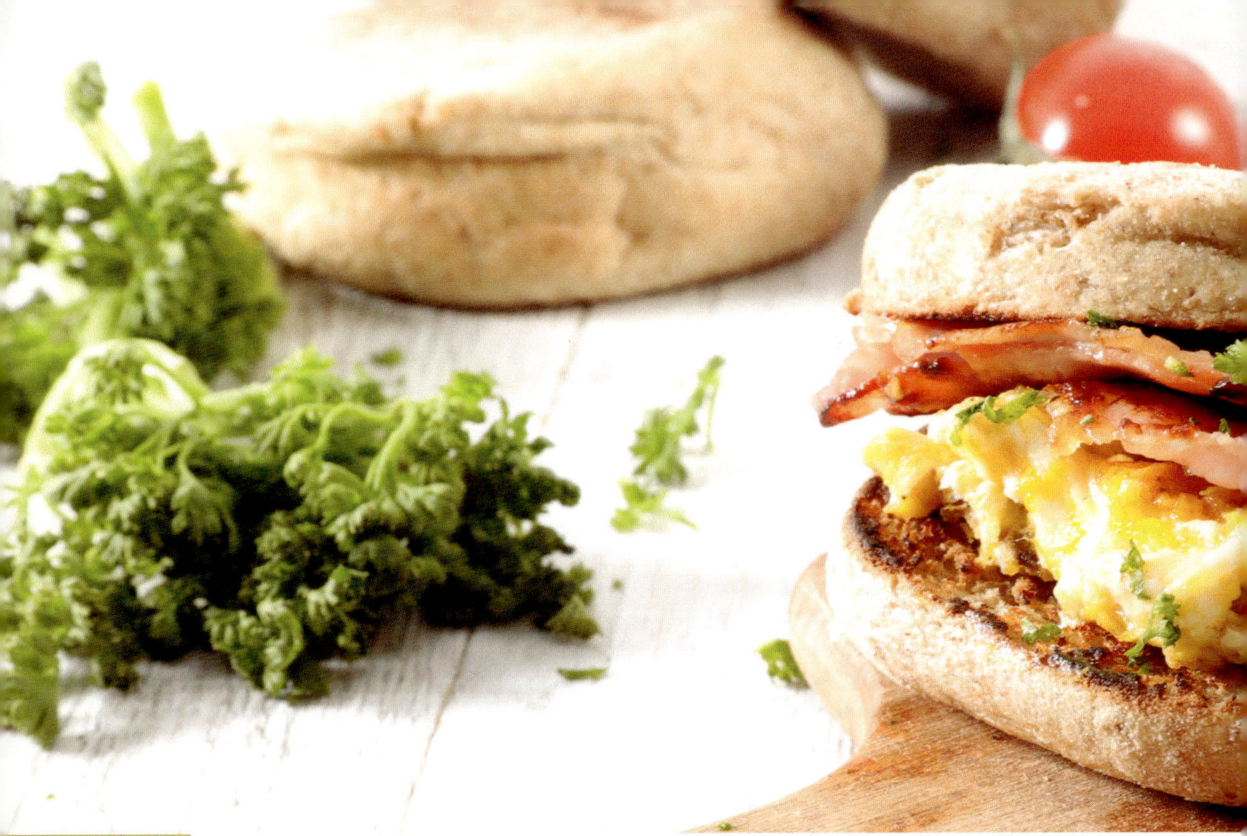

Ham, cheese and tomato muffin

SERVES
1

A simple breakfast to grab in one hand as you're walking out the door.

Options

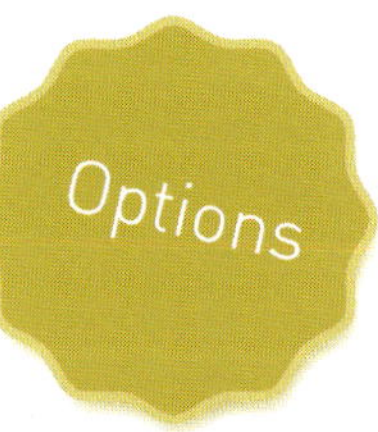

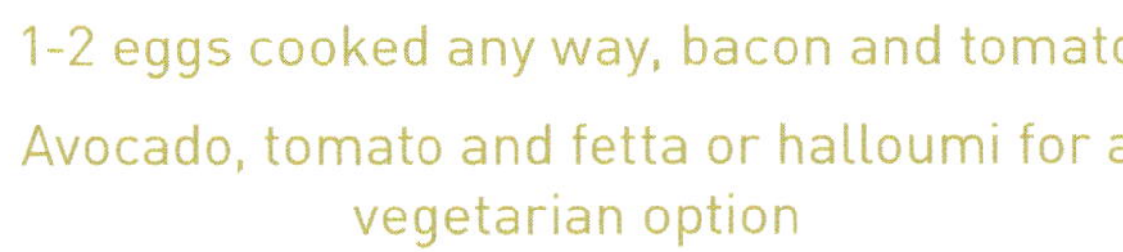

1-2 eggs cooked any way, bacon and tomato

Avocado, tomato and fetta or halloumi for a vegetarian option

This can also be done with sliced bread or wrap.

BREAKFAST

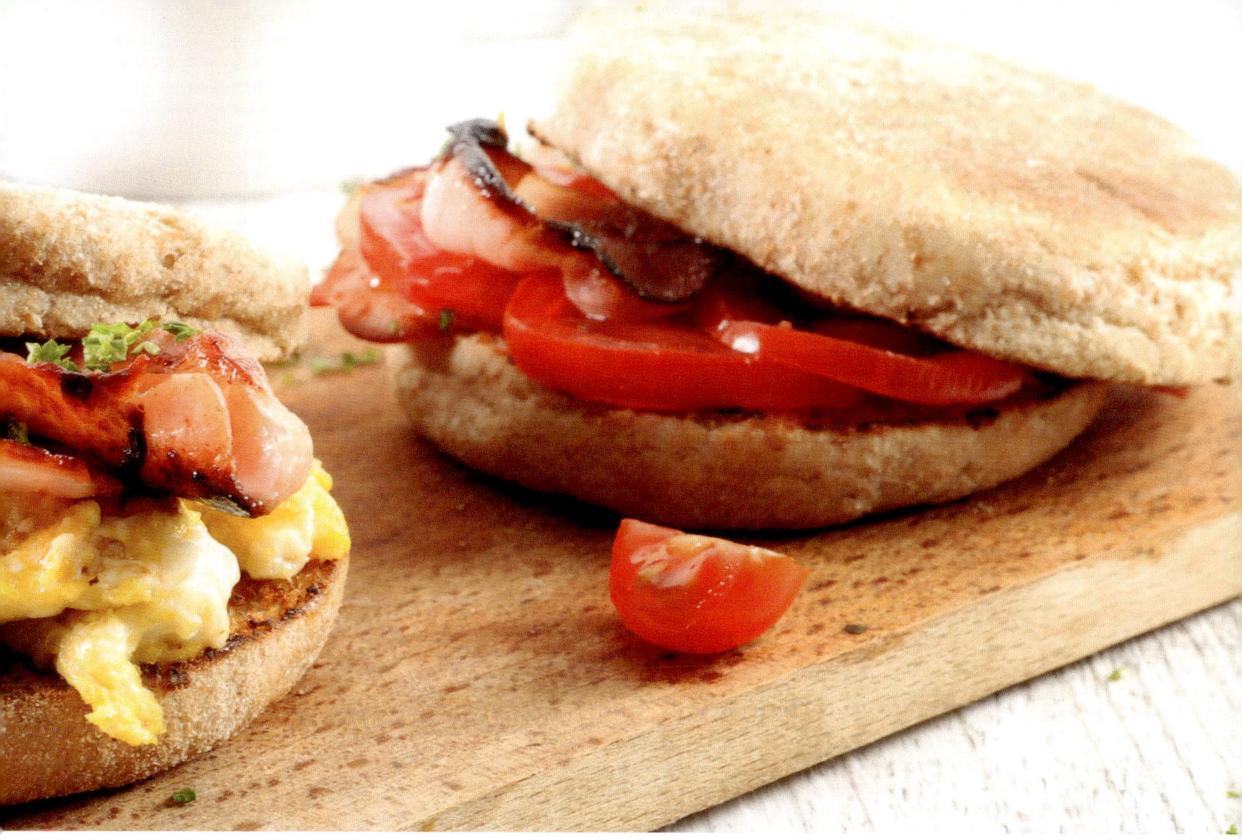

Ingredients

Wholemeal or wholegrain English muffins packet (gluten free also available at supermarket)

2-3 slices ham or 2-3 short-cut bacon pieces

1 slice low-fat tasty cheese

½ sliced tomato

Method

1. If using bacon, cook in pan
2. Place ham/bacon, cheese and tomato on one side of muffin (fresh or toasted)
3. Optional: add avocado to other side
4. Place pieces together like a sandwich and enjoy.

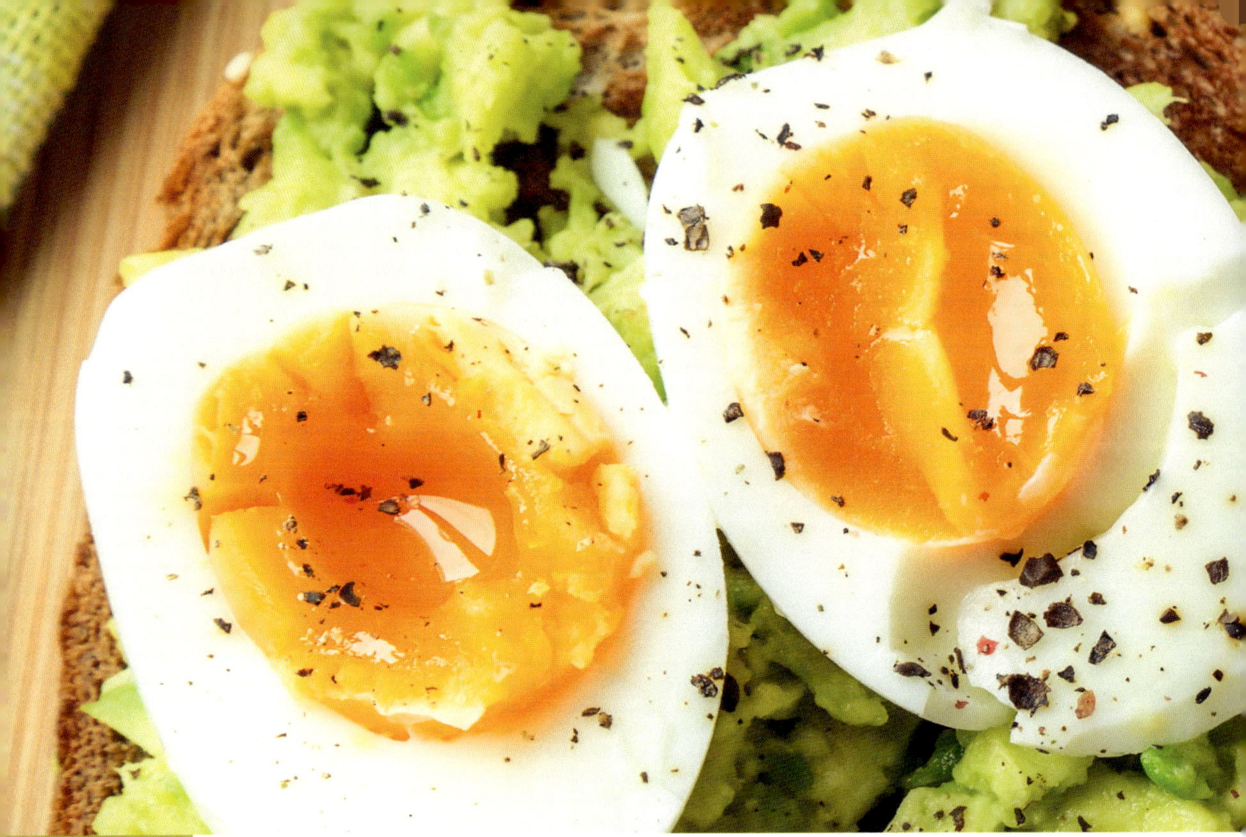

Avocado on toast

SERVES
1

The classic avo smash that you pay considerably for at a café can be made at home for a fraction of the price.

Options

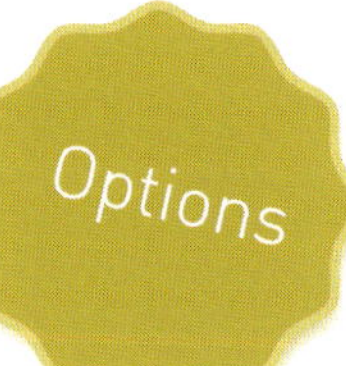

Get creative with your base.

Try sweet potato slices, rice cakes, paleo seeded bread, seeded crackers or a bed of leftover cooked greens.

BREAKFAST

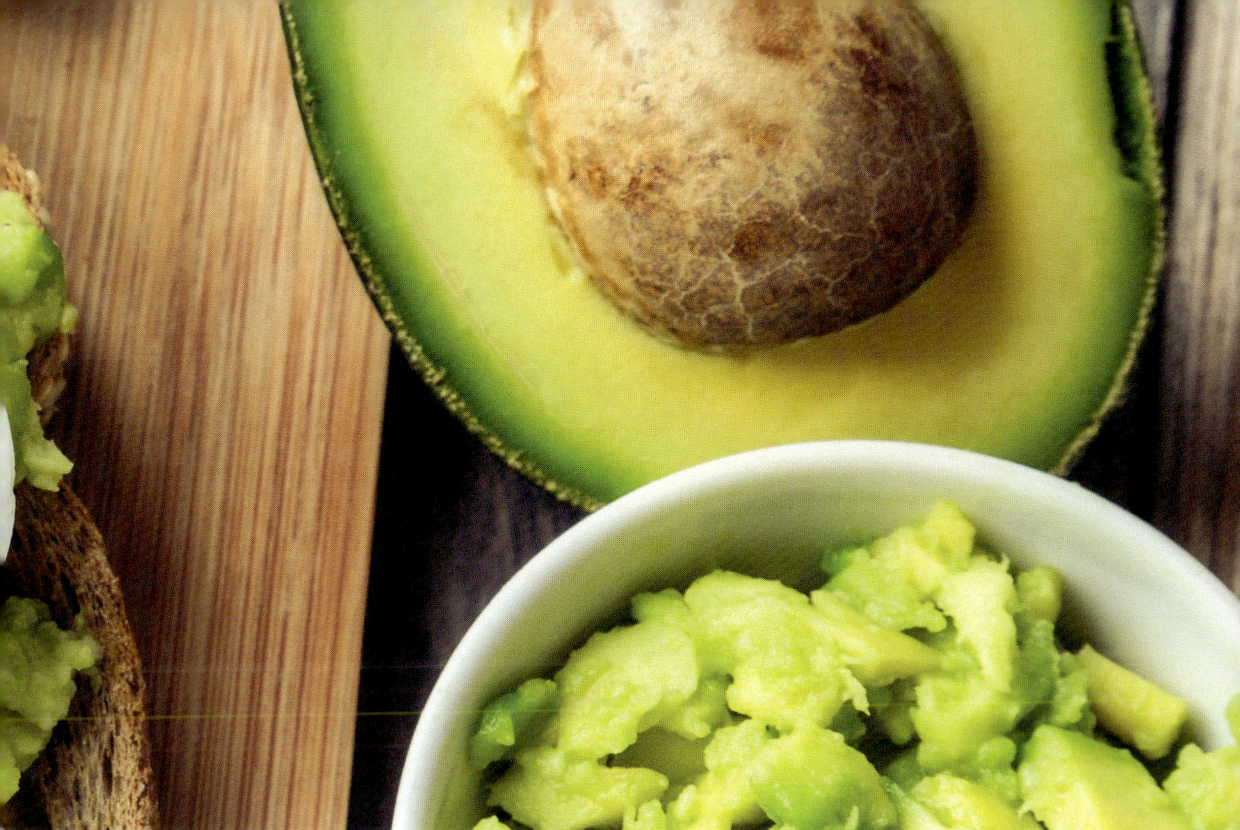

Ingredients

1 slice of toast of choice

¼–½ avocado

1 egg cooked (poached or hard boiled)

¼ lime

Other toppings of choice: chilli flakes, tomato, fetta, dukkah, flaked almonds, or salt and pepper

Method

1. Toast bread
2. Slice or mash avocado on the toast
3. Add poached/hard boiled egg
4. Add a squeeze of lime and topping of choice.

Eggs plus sides

SERVES
1

Creativity at its best! A bowl of goodness with all your faves.

Eggs are so versatile and easy to prepare.

You can have them poached/boiled/fried/scrambled/as an omelette or in a frittata

Add a side and breakfast couldn't be simpler.

Ingredients

2-3 eggs

Spinach

Mushrooms

Avocado

10 chopped almonds

Tomatoes

Salmon slices

Crumbled fetta

Method

1. Place eggs cooked any way and avocado in a bowl
2. Add sides of choice
3. Aim for two proteins + three veggies + avocado.

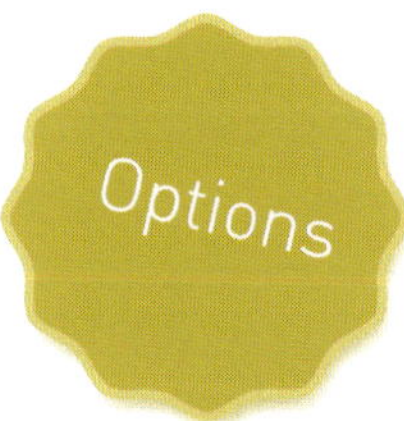

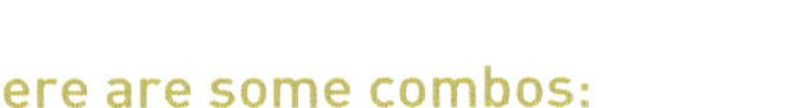

Scrambled eggs and spinach with mushrooms, tomatoes and crumbled fetta

Poached eggs on a bed of spinach with a side of salmon, avocado and crushed nuts.

BREAKFAST

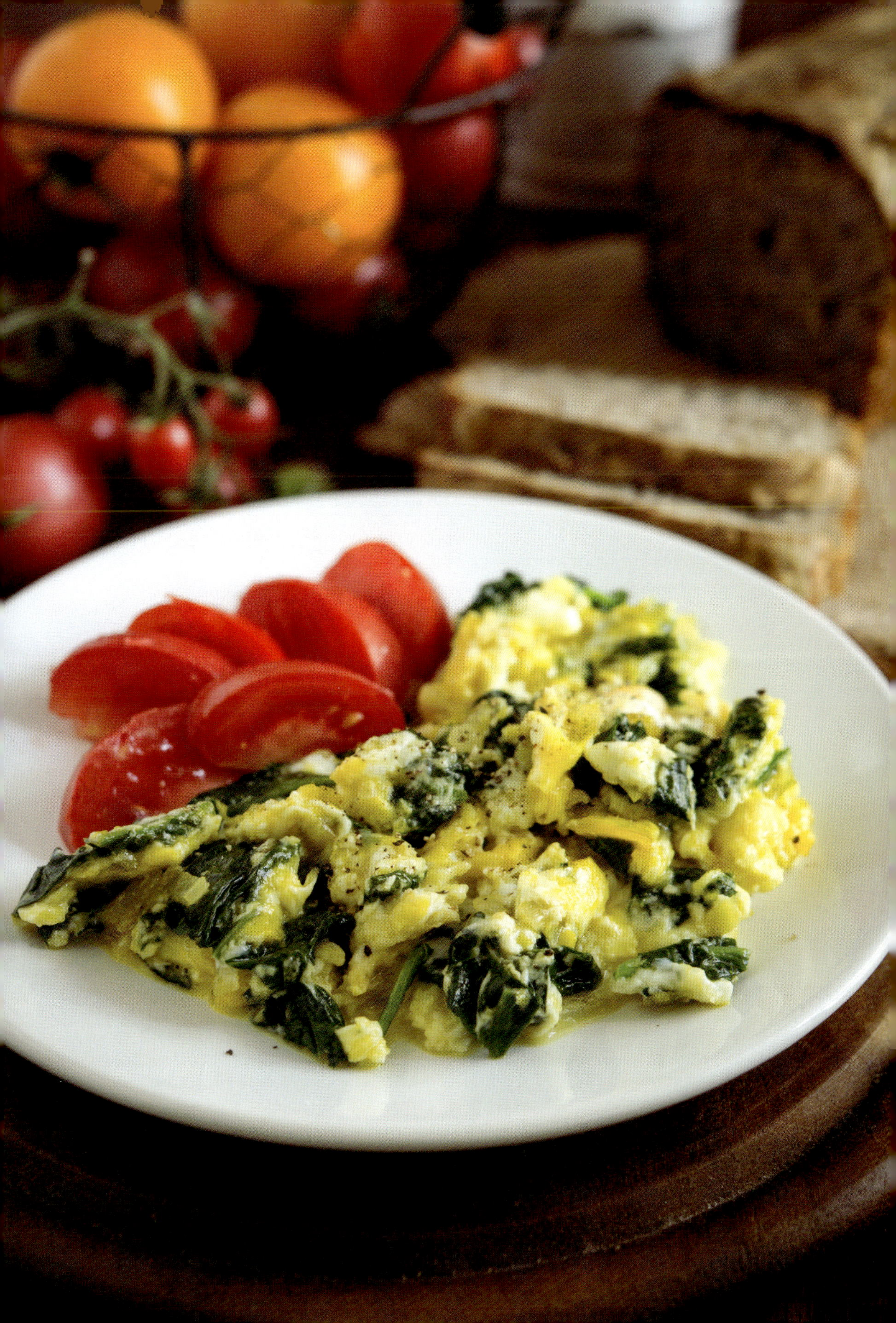

Fritters

SERVES
3

Ingredients

4 cups grated zucchini

¼ cup almond meal

3 tablespoons grated parmesan

3 eggs

½ red capsicum or grated carrot

1 cup corn kernels

Salt and pepper

Olive oil for cooking

Method

1. Grate the zucchini
2. Squeeze out all the moisture from the zucchini with your hands
3. Place all ingredients in a bowl. Mix well until combined
4. Add a touch more almond meal if needed to hold shape
5. Cook fritters in a pan over a medium heat in a little olive oil for 2 minutes each side
6. This makes about 10 fritters. Great to serve with a rocket and fetta salad or avocado and tomato salsa.

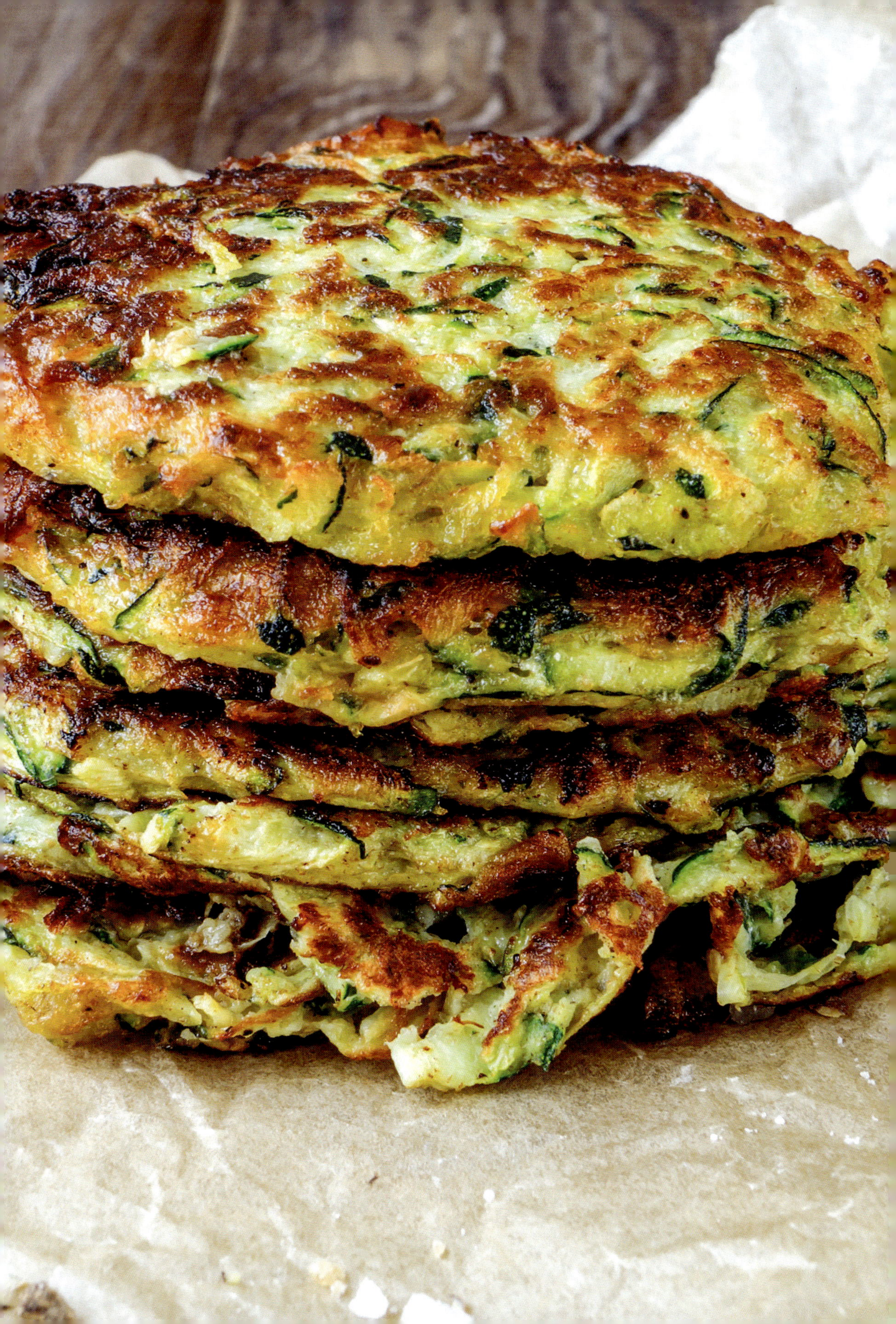

Peanut butter/almond spread on toast

with sliced banana and cinnamon

SERVES
1

A fave with the kids and the adults.

Ingredients

1 slice of toast

100% peanut butter/ almond spread

Sliced banana

Cinnamon for dusting (optional)

Method

1. Spread approx. 1 tablespoon of your preferred spread on warm toast
2. Top with banana circles and a dusting of cinnamon.

Great on rice cakes/Vita-Weats/crispbreads and crackers too.

BREAKFAST

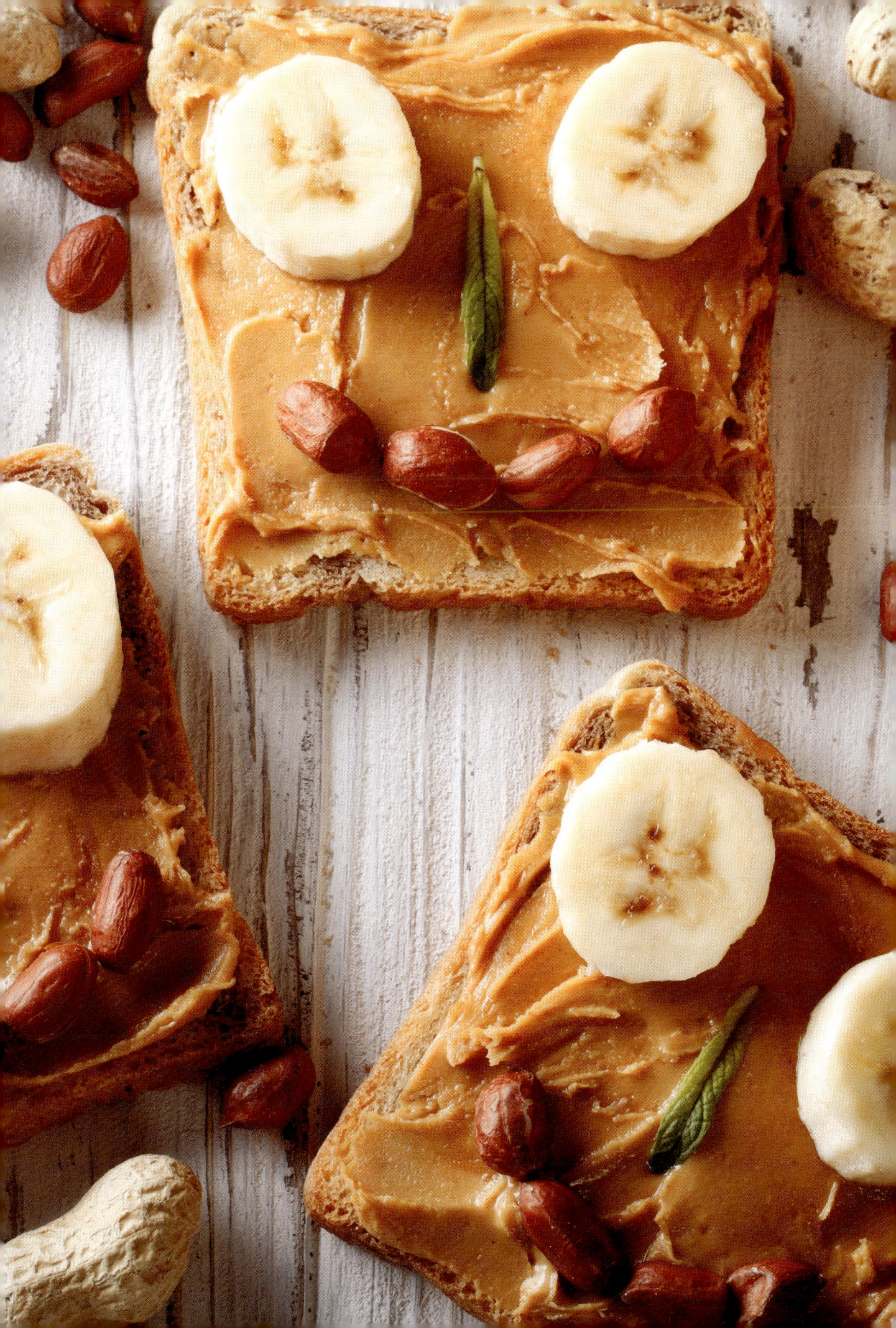

Smoothie

SERVES
1

With a blender this can be a quick breakfast you can have on the go.

Bananas contain potassium and B vitamins which boost energy levels, so a great start to the day.

Ingredients

1 frozen banana

½ teaspoon honey (optional)

½ cup almond milk/milk of choice

¼ cup water

1 cup ice cubes

Dusting of cinnamon

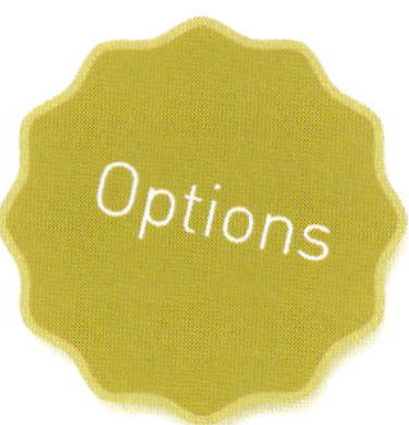

Berry Boost – This smoothie is packed full of antioxidants and vitamin C Replace banana and cinnamon with ¾ cup mixed berries

Coffee Crazy – A great drink before or after a workout. A powerful breakfast with an energy boost. Replace honey with a single shot of espresso coffee or 1.5 teaspoons instant coffee

For the growing boys – Add 1-2 tablespoon oats

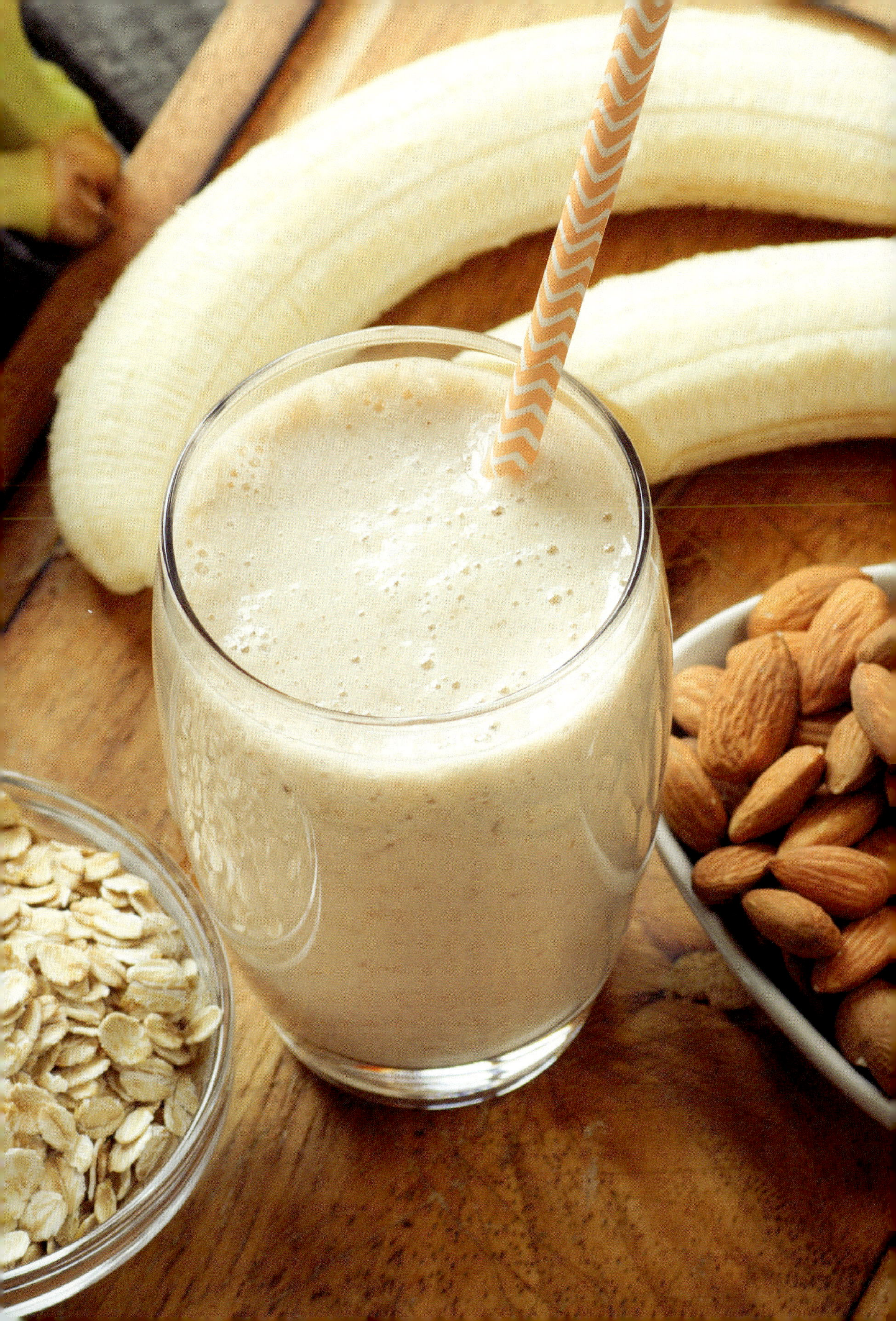

Homemade grain-free muesli

MAKES
Bulk

Ingredients

¼ cup natural activated buckinis

¼ cup almond meal

¼ cup shredded coconut

¼ cup of each – brazil nut, pecan, almonds, walnuts, pistachios

¼ cup of sunflower seeds

¼ cup pepita seeds

1 teaspoon each – flaxseed, sesame seed

1 tablespoon ground cinnamon

¼ cup goji berries (optional)

½ cup plain oats (optional grain)

Method

1. Place meal, buckinis, coconut and cinnamon in container and stir
2. Chop all nuts and add to coconut mixture
3. Add seeds, goji berries and stir, adding more cinnamon to liking.

Great with a few slices of banana, a drizzle of honey and almond milk.

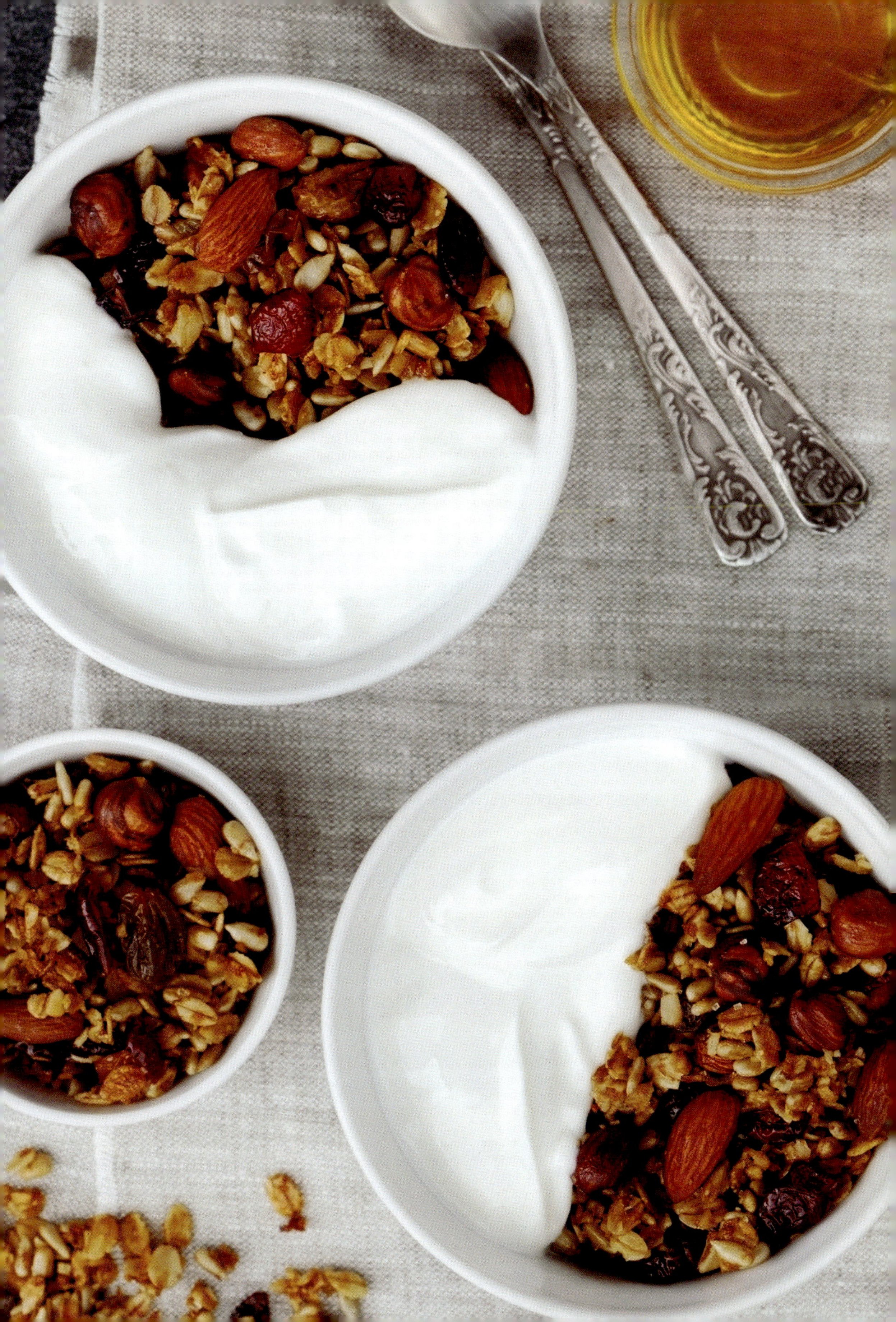

Granola

MAKES
Bulk

Ingredients

1½ cup raw oats

¼ cup shredded coconut

¼ cup chopped walnuts

¼ cup flaked almonds

¼ cup mixed pepitas and sunflower seeds

2 tablespoons chia

2 tablespoons sesame seeds

1 tablespoon cinnamon

2 egg whites

2 tablespoons raw honey

Method

1. Place all dry ingredients in bowl and mix with a spoon
2. Add two egg whites and 2 tablespoons of just melted raw honey
3. Bake in oven on baking paper for 30 minutes on low–medium heat (160°C) until golden
4. Allow to cool and store in airtight container.

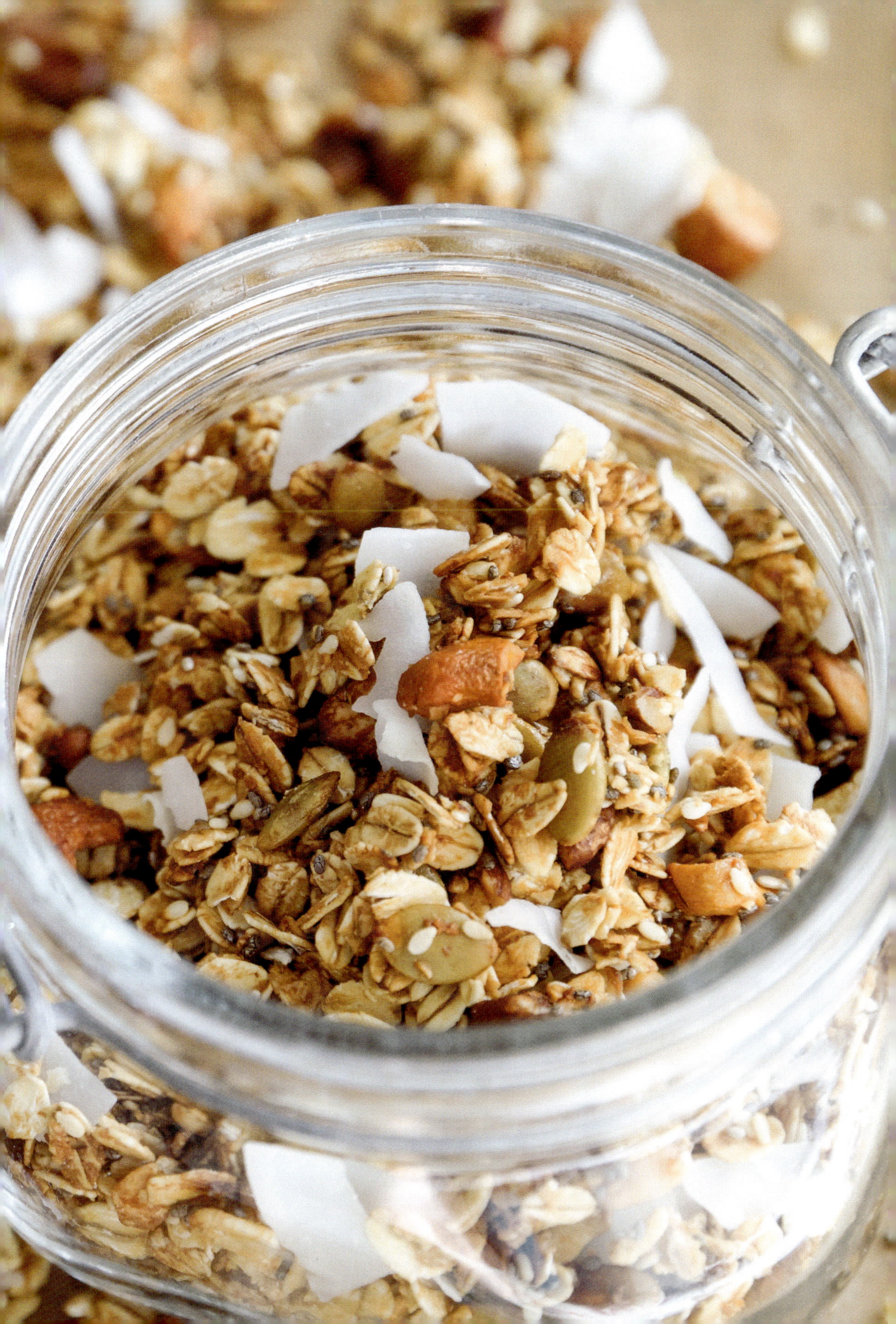

Yoghurt and fruit cups

SERVES
1

A quick breakfast or snack that the kids can do without any help. Let them choose their favourite fruits and muesli to create a masterpiece.

This recipe also makes a great dessert and can be presented in a jar for entertaining.

Use fruits in season and allow your creativity to shine.

Ingredients

½ cup plain fruit-free yoghurt

½ cup of any fruit sliced/chopped

½ cup muesli
(see earlier recipes)

Jar for serving

Honey, nuts and seeds
for topping

Grated dark chocolate flakes
(optional)

Method

1. Layer jar with muesli/fruit/ yoghurt then repeat
2. Finish with fruit on top
3. Add your nuts and seeds, a drizzle honey or some grated dark chocolate.

BREAKFAST

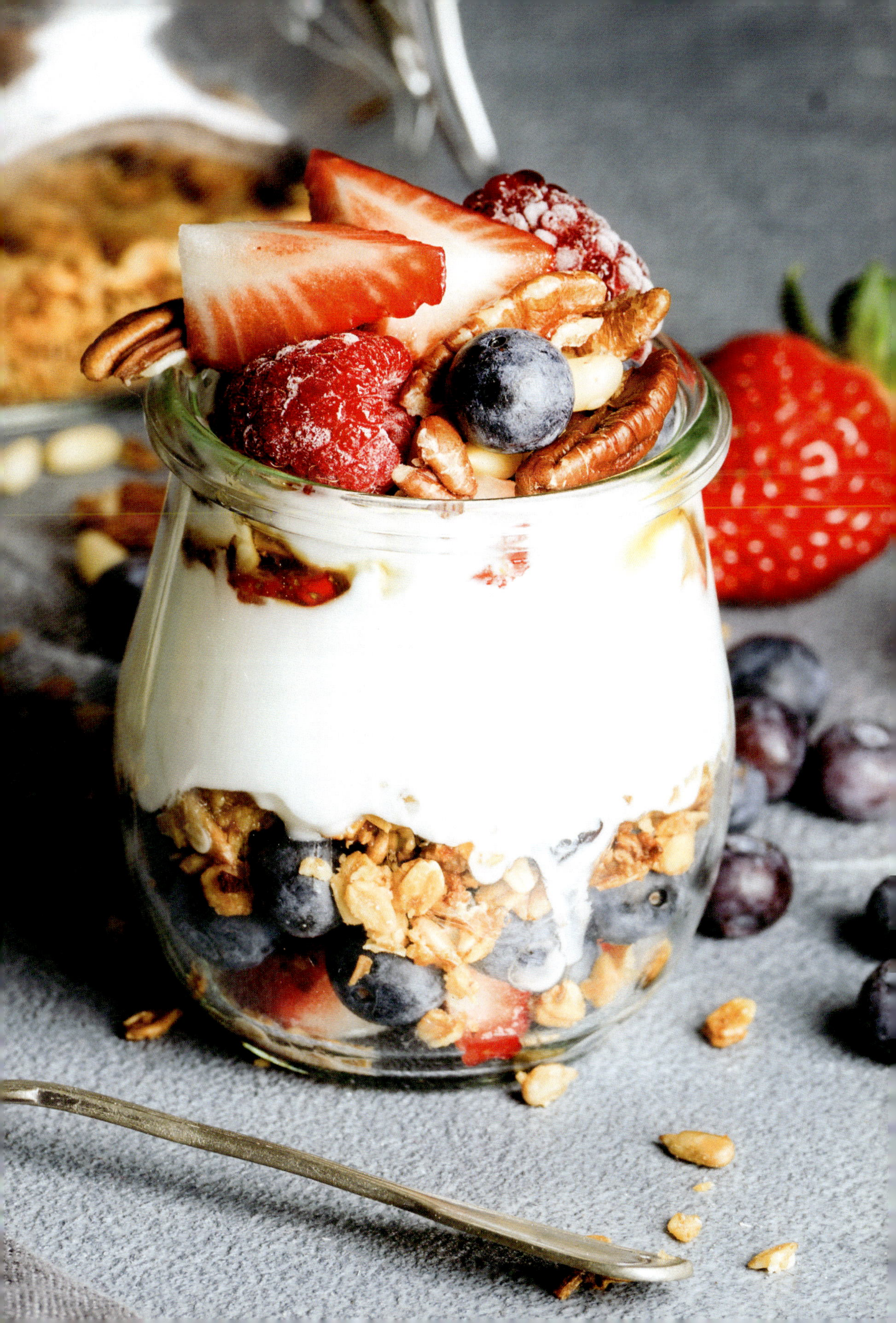

Buckwheat pancakes

SERVES
2

Ingredients

150ml milk

60g buckwheat flour

60g almond meal

½ teaspoon baking soda

1 teaspoon apple cider vinegar

Method

1. Mix the milk, buckwheat flour and almond meal in a bowl to a smooth batter
2. Add the baking soda and vinegar and mix well
3. Melt 1 tablespoon of butter or coconut oil in a heavy-based, non- stick pan and add 2 tablespoons of the batter at a time to make small pancakes
4. Cook for a couple of minutes on each side.

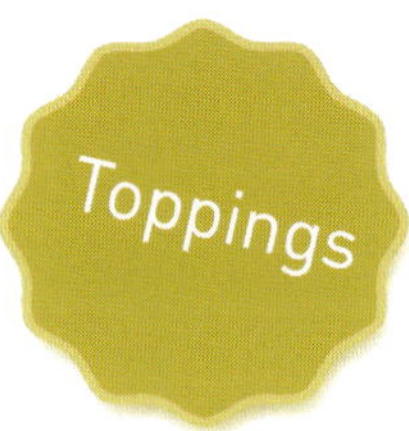

Toppings you can add to the pancakes include:

A spread of a soft cheese such as Brie with sliced tomato and chopped spinach

Sliced banana for a sweet flavour. Experiment with your favourite healthy toppings.

BREAKFAST

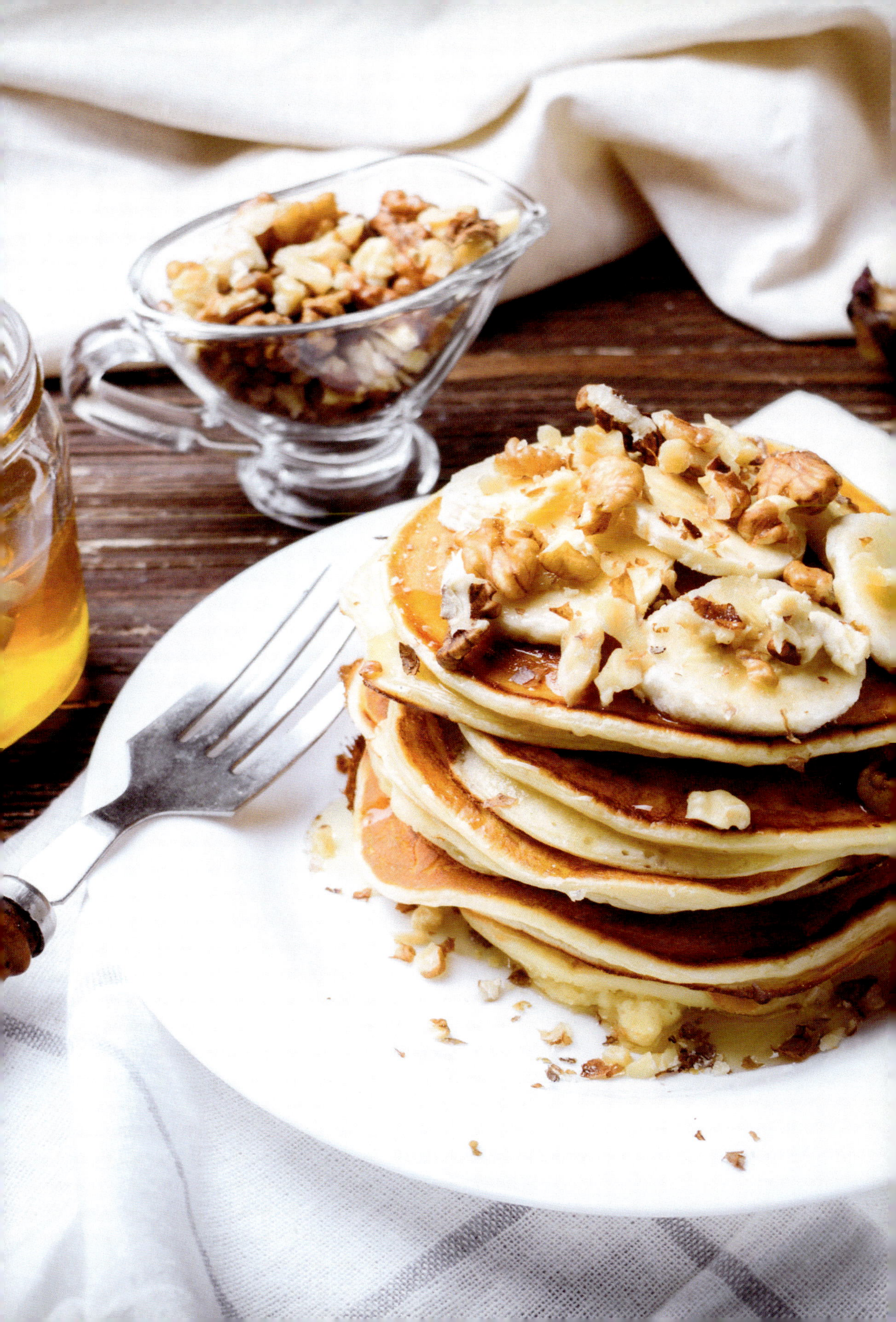

Egg muffins

MAKES
10

Great for a portable breakfast, morning or afternoon tea or when still hungry.

Ingredients

12 eggs whisked

¾ cup of chopped mushroom, spinach and red capsicum

Or any veggies you would like to add

¾ cup cubed fetta

Method

1. Whisk 12 eggs
2. Place pre-cooked mushroom, spinach, capsicum, salt and pepper in medium-sized muffin trays
3. Can add herbs and spices to taste – parsley etc
4. Cover veggies with beaten egg and fetta cubes
5. Bake at 160°C for about 30 minutes or until cooked and golden.

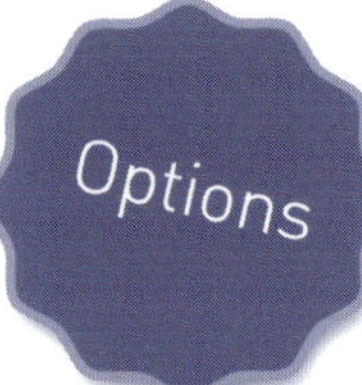

Add ham, bacon, grated cheese or any filling you may have

Kids love the bacon and grated cheese

All these variations make a great frittata by baking in a deep dish.

SNACKS

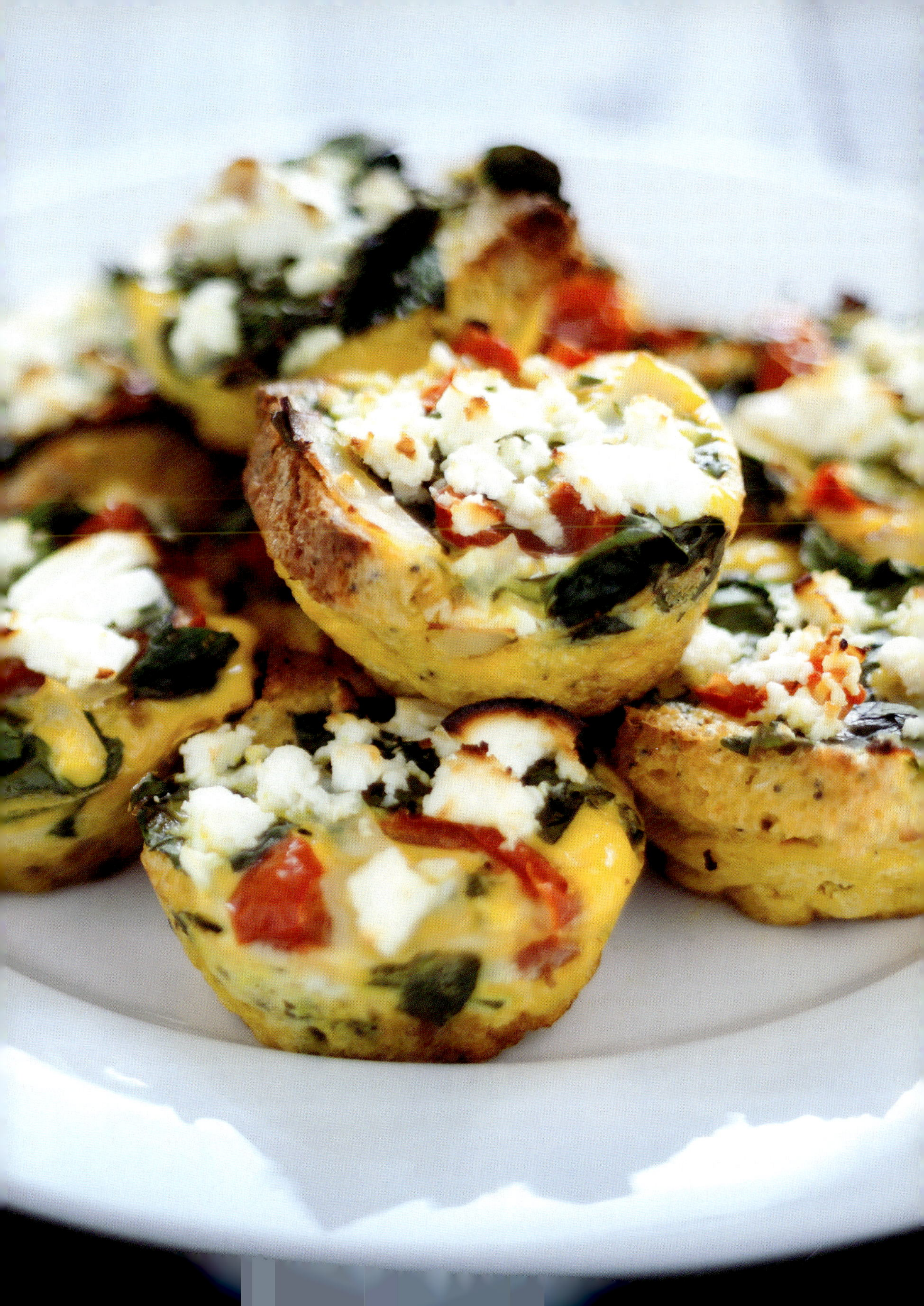

Frittata

SERVES
2

Make this in a baking dish and slice into portions with a side salad.

Ingredients

250g pumpkin chopped

10g butter

1 garlic clove, finely chopped

2 leeks chopped

5 eggs

Small bunch asparagus

Method

1. Preheat oven to 200°C
2. Trim ends of asparagus and cook in boiling water for 1 minute
3. Place pumpkin on a baking tray. Drizzle with olive oil and season. Roast for 6 minutes.
4. Reduce oven to 180°C
5. Heat the butter in a pan. Add garlic and leek and cook for a few minutes
6. Lightly beat eggs in a bowl and season
7. Layer pumpkin, leek and asparagus in a pan/dish. Pour the egg mixture into the pan
8. Cook in the oven for 20 minutes or until cooked through.

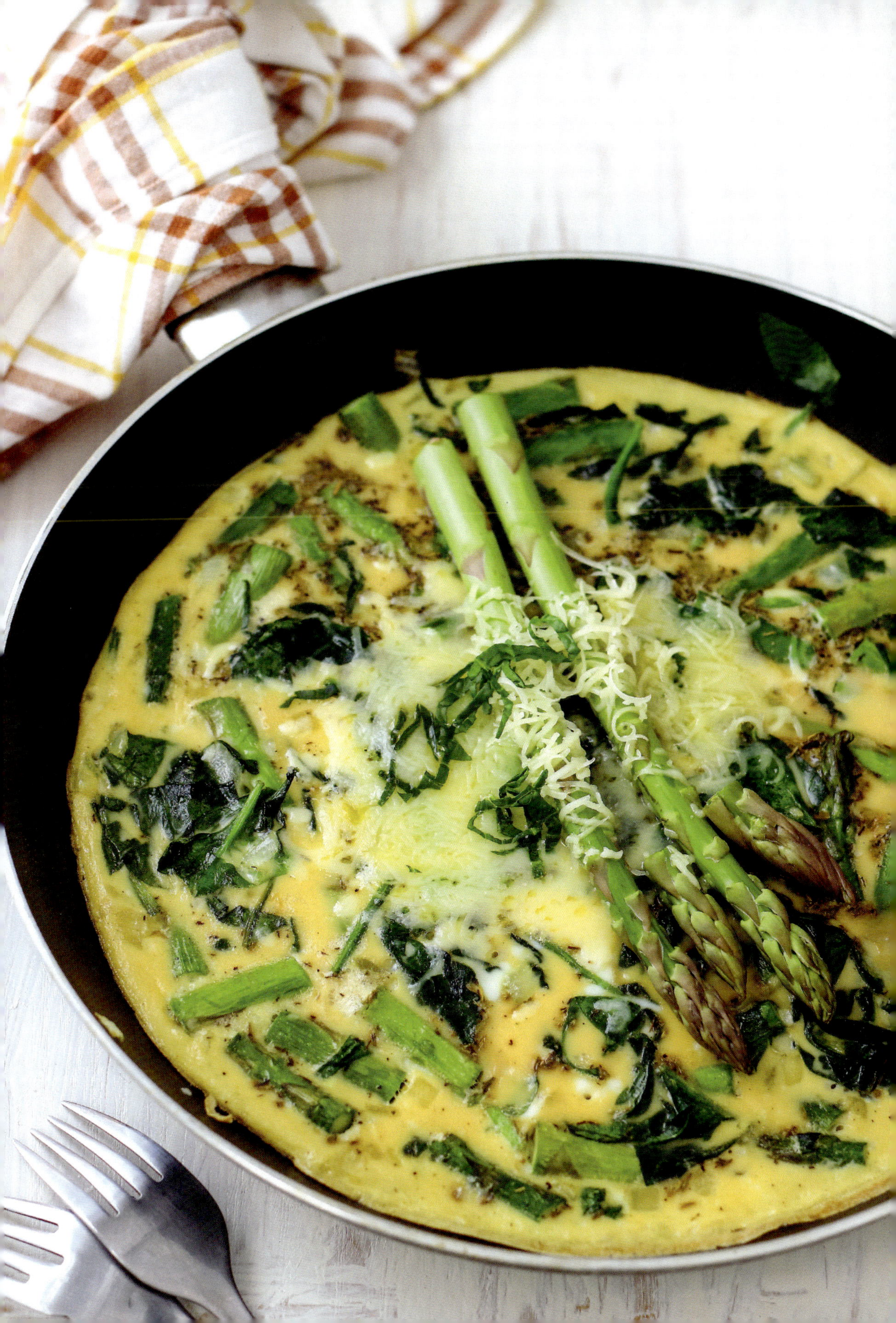

Basic bone broth

MAKES
1 Litre

Enjoy straight away while hot or keep in fridge or freezer to use as homemade stock that can be added to casseroles, soups and stews.

Ingredients

3-4 chicken carcasses

2 onions roughly chopped

4 crushed garlic cloves

½ bunch of chopped celery

2 tablespoons good quality sea salt

3 sprigs of thyme

1 litre water

1 tablespoon apple cider vinegar

Method

1. Combine chicken carcass, water onion, garlic, celery, thyme, salt and apple cider vinegar into a slow cooker or pressure cooker
2. Slow cook for 24 hours, or pressure cook for 1½ hours until bones have broken down
3. Drain the contents through a sieve to extract the liquid.

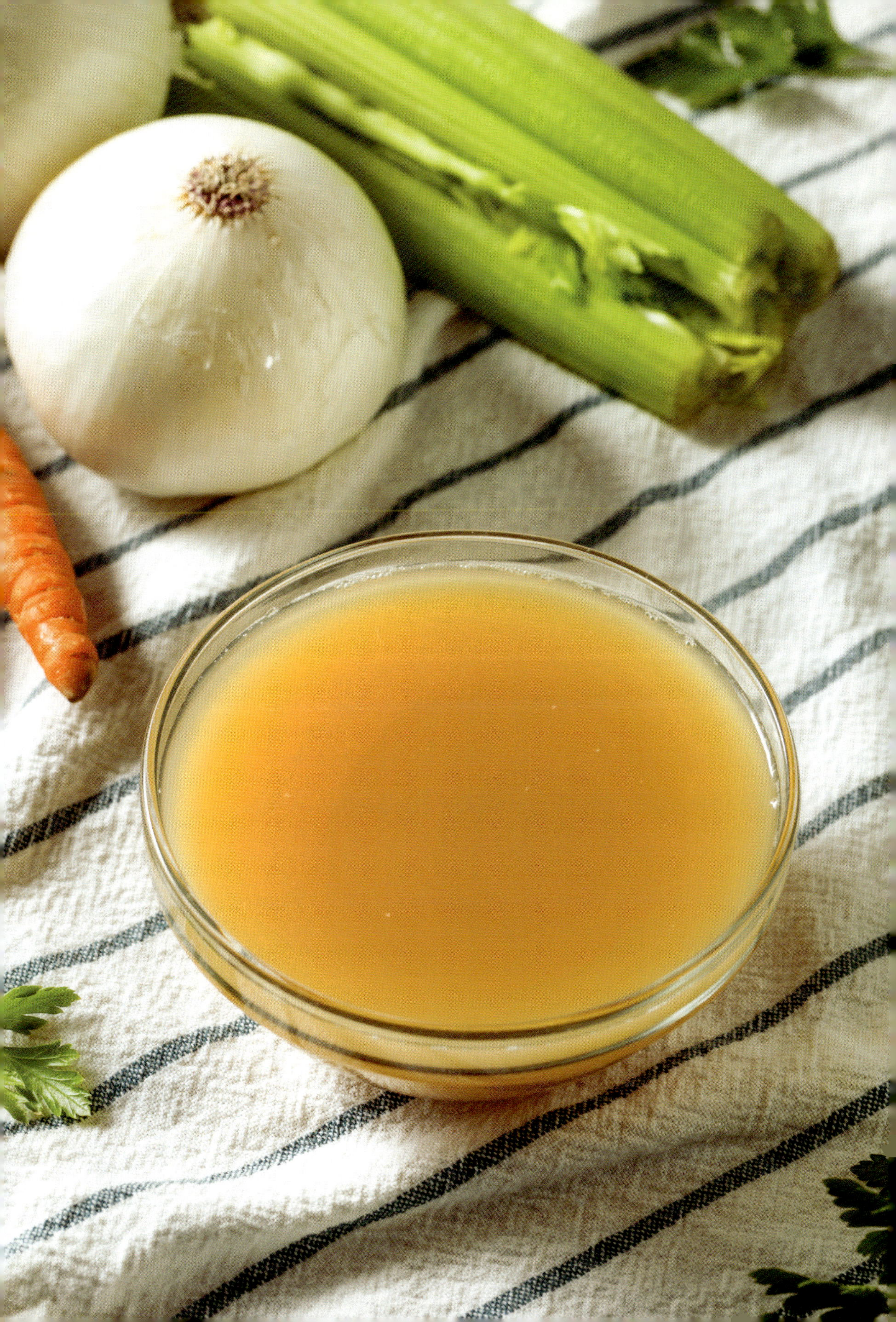

Raw veggie sticks

with avocado smash, hommus or boiled eggs

SERVES
2

Ingredients

2 boiled eggs cut in half

1 carrot

1 cucumber

1 celery stick

¾ red capsicum

1 avocado for avo smash

Juice of ½ a lime

Hommus – see recipe on page 82 or use pre-made pots found in the supermarket. Remember to check the ingredients lists for the unnecessary stuff.

Method

1. Chop veggies into 6cm strips
2. Make avocado smash – combine 1 mashed avocado with juice of lemon or lime, salt and pepper
3. Combine onto serving plate and enjoy.

This makes a great entertaining platter with some fresh fruit, nuts and seeds.

Variation: Try hommus instead of the avocado smash.

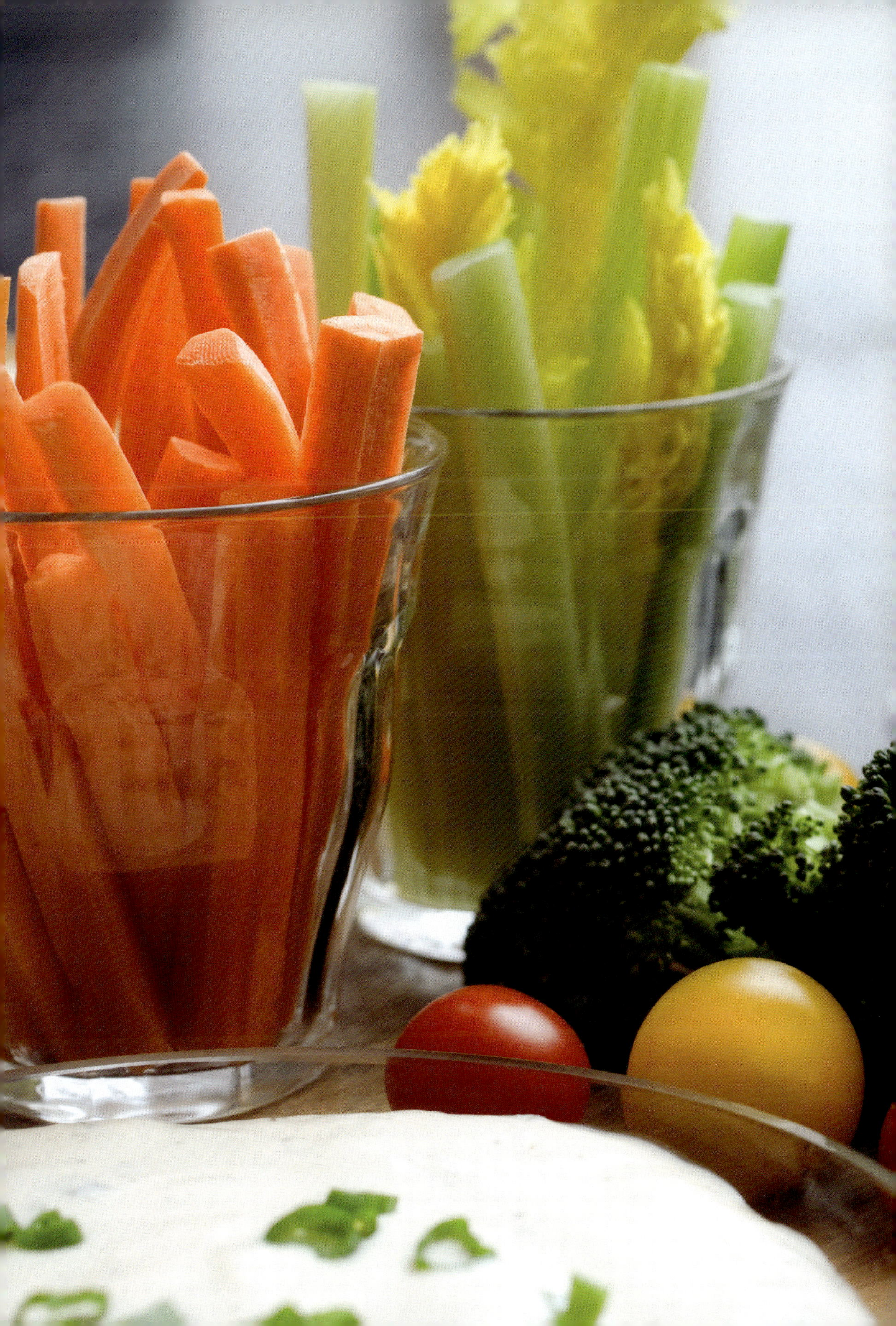

Homemade humus

SERVES
2-4

Ingredients

1 cup dried chickpeas

1 clove garlic finely chopped

1 tablespoon tahini

2 tablespoons olive oil

juice of half a lemon

Celtic sea salt and pepper to taste

Method

1. Soak chickpeas overnight in filtered water

2. Blend chickpeas then add garlic, tahini, lemon juice and olive oil. Add more olive oil if necessary to make a smoother consistency.

3. Season with salt and pepper. Serve in a bowl (optional – drizzle with olive oil and sprinkle with paprika).

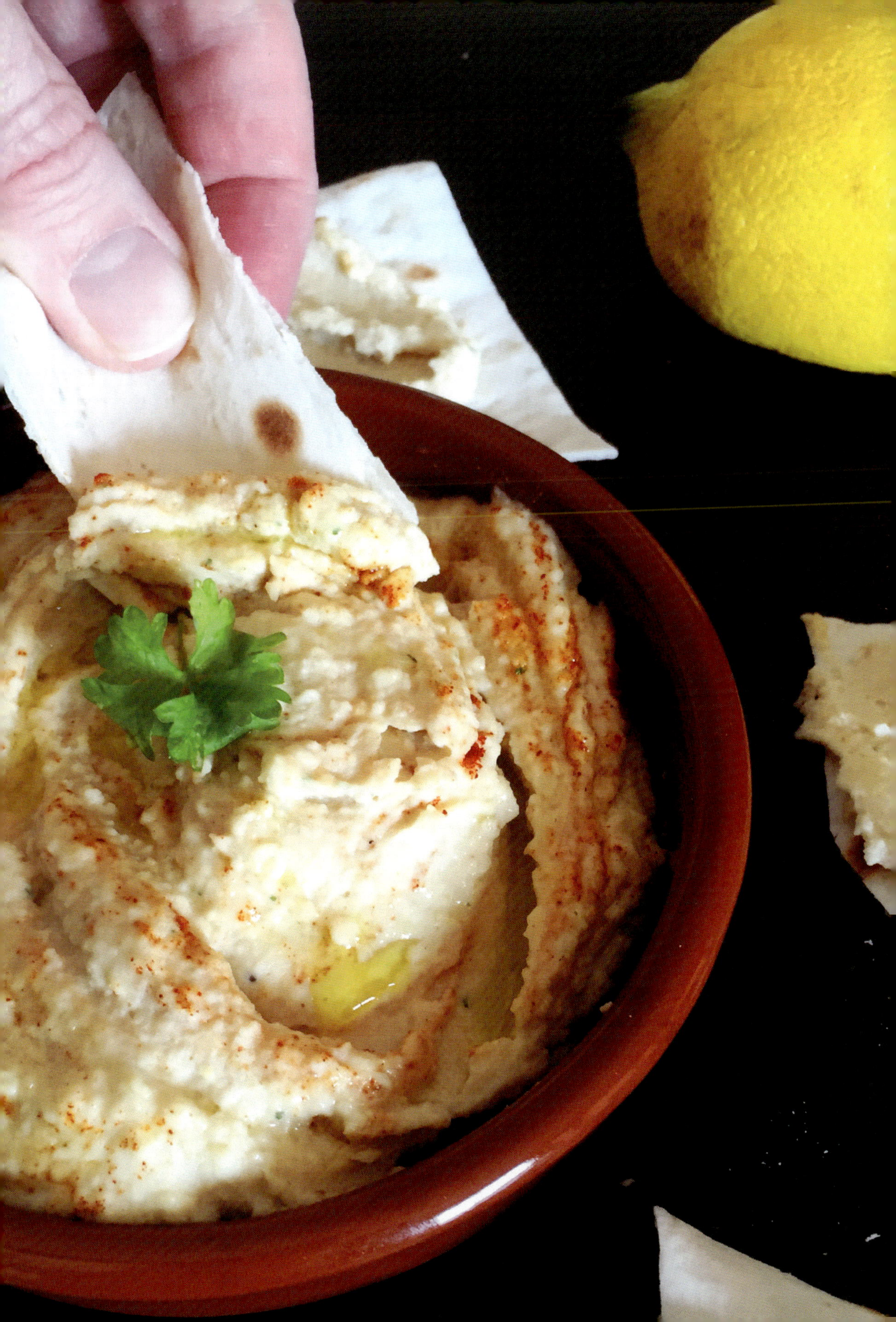

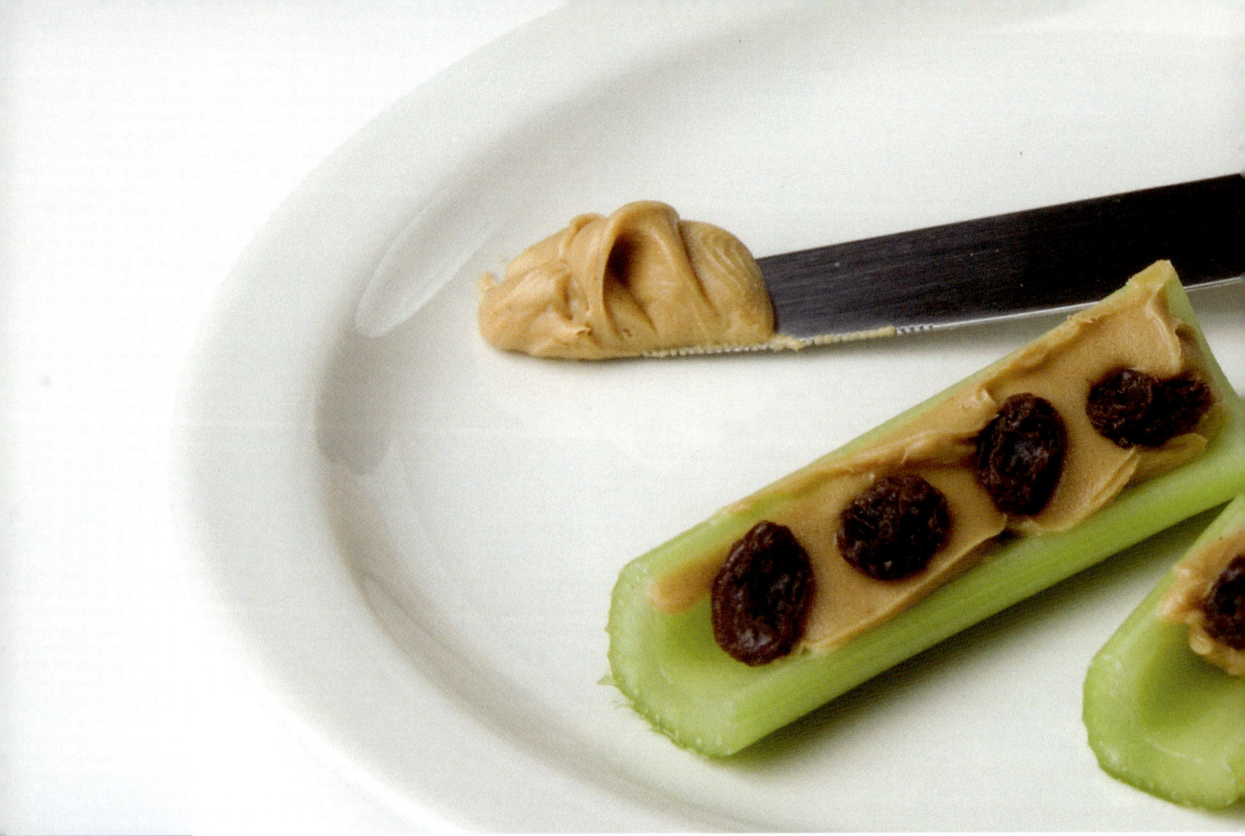

Celery boats

SERVES
1

A great way to add a serve of veggies to your day.

Options

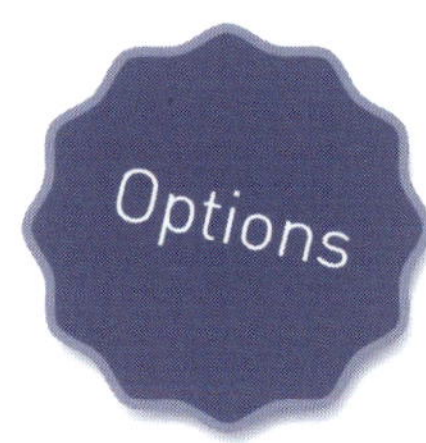

You can use cottage cheese, grated cheese, spreadable fetta, mashed avo or hommus.

SNACKS

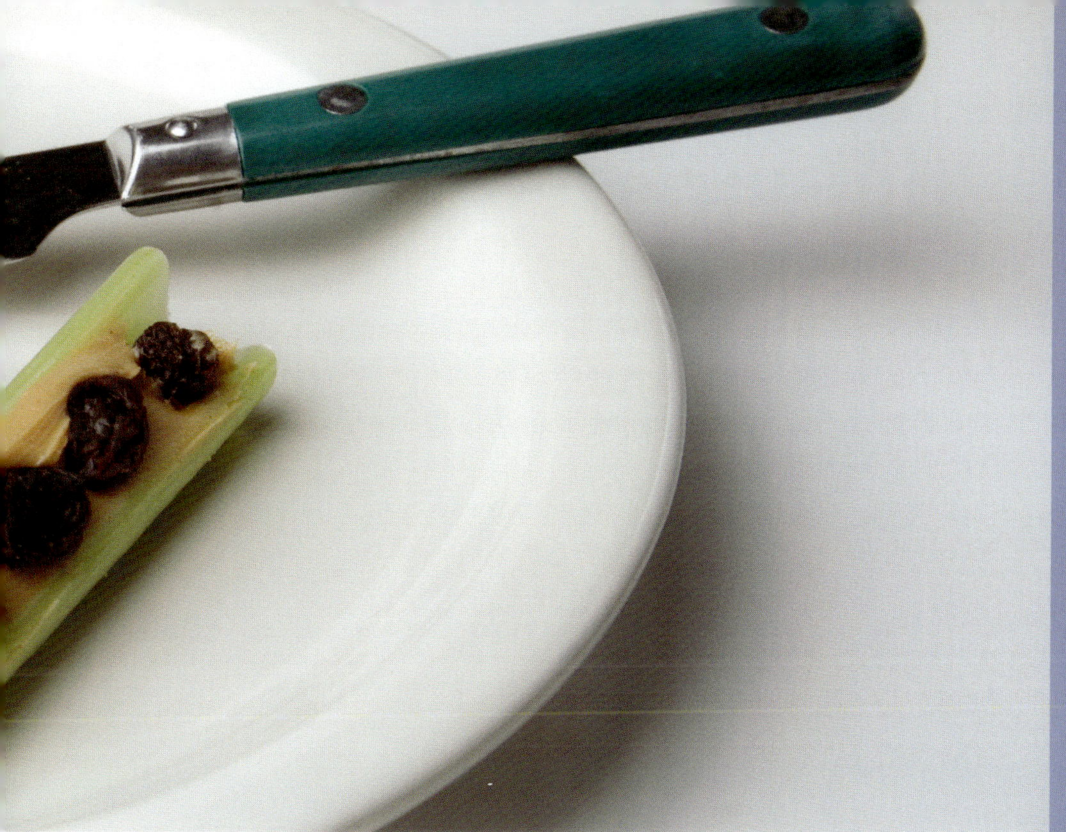

Ingredients

4 celery sticks about 10cm long

Your choice of peanut butter/ spreadable cheese/other toppings

Method

1. Wash and cut celery into 10cm pieces
2. Spread peanut butter and top with something fun such as sultanas, flaked almonds or even a few choc chips.

Nut and seed crackers

For low-carb enthusiasts, seeded crackers are the way to go.

There are some readily available at the supermarket or you can make your own.

Use an avocado smash, nut spread, cheese or hommus as an accompaniment.

MAKES
6

Ingredients

1 cup almonds

½ cup flaxseeds

½ cup filtered water

2 teaspoons olive oil

¼ teaspoon salt

For a perfect platter arrange these with dip of your choice, fruit, nuts and veggie sticks.

Method

1 Line oven tray with baking paper

2 Blend flaxseeds and almonds to fine meal

3 Mix oil and salt into mixture. Add water until it's a thick consistency

4 Roll out thinly between 2 sheet of baking paper, remove top sheet and put onto the oven tray

5 Bake for 1½ hours at 70°C. Turn the heat down to 40°C and bake for another 5 hours.

6 Turn the large cracker over and bake for a further 5 hours

7 You are dehydrating the nuts (rather than cooking) at a very low heat. That's why it takes so long. If you have a dehydrator, use that rather than the oven. When ready, break the cracker into smaller pieces and store in an airtight container.

Tuna, corn, and rice

SERVES
1

A simple yet satisfying snack or meal for a hungry child.

This makes a great meal for before or after a workout.

Often when my eldest comes home from training she is exhausted and hungry. This is a great mix of carbs and protein to satisfy hunger and to help her recover.

Ingredients

½ cup cooked rice

1 small tin corn drained

1 tin tuna drained

Method

Mix all ingredients together and season as needed with salt, pepper, lime juice or herbs.

Popcorn

SERVES
1

A very simple high-fibre snack that can involve the kids too.

Ingredients

1 packet of organic popping corn, using as much as needed for 2 cups of cooked popcorn

Method

1. Place organic corn in a saucepan with a teaspoon of butter on low with the lid on, or in a popcorn machine if you have one
2. Within minutes you have fresh, warm salt and butter-free popcorn!

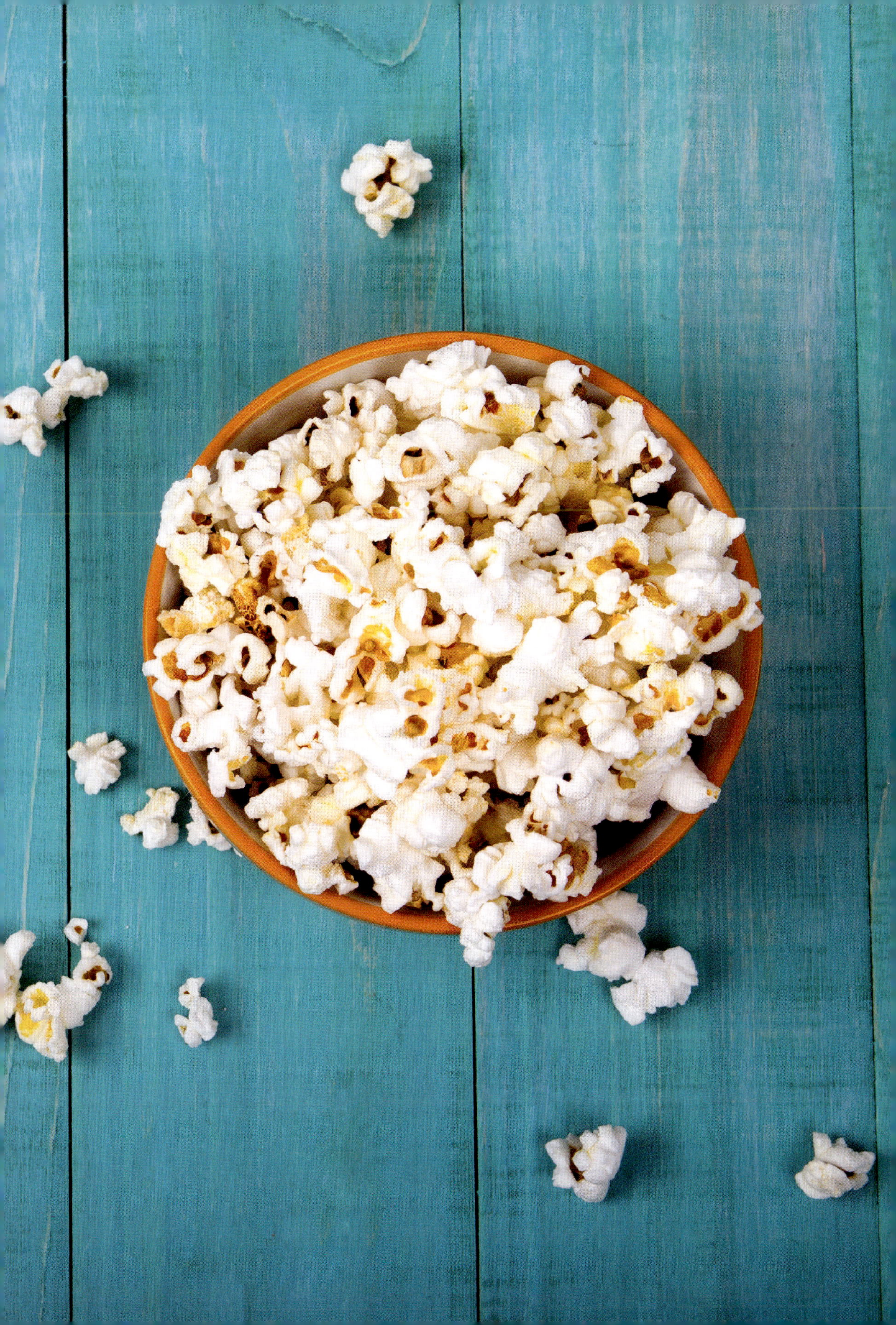

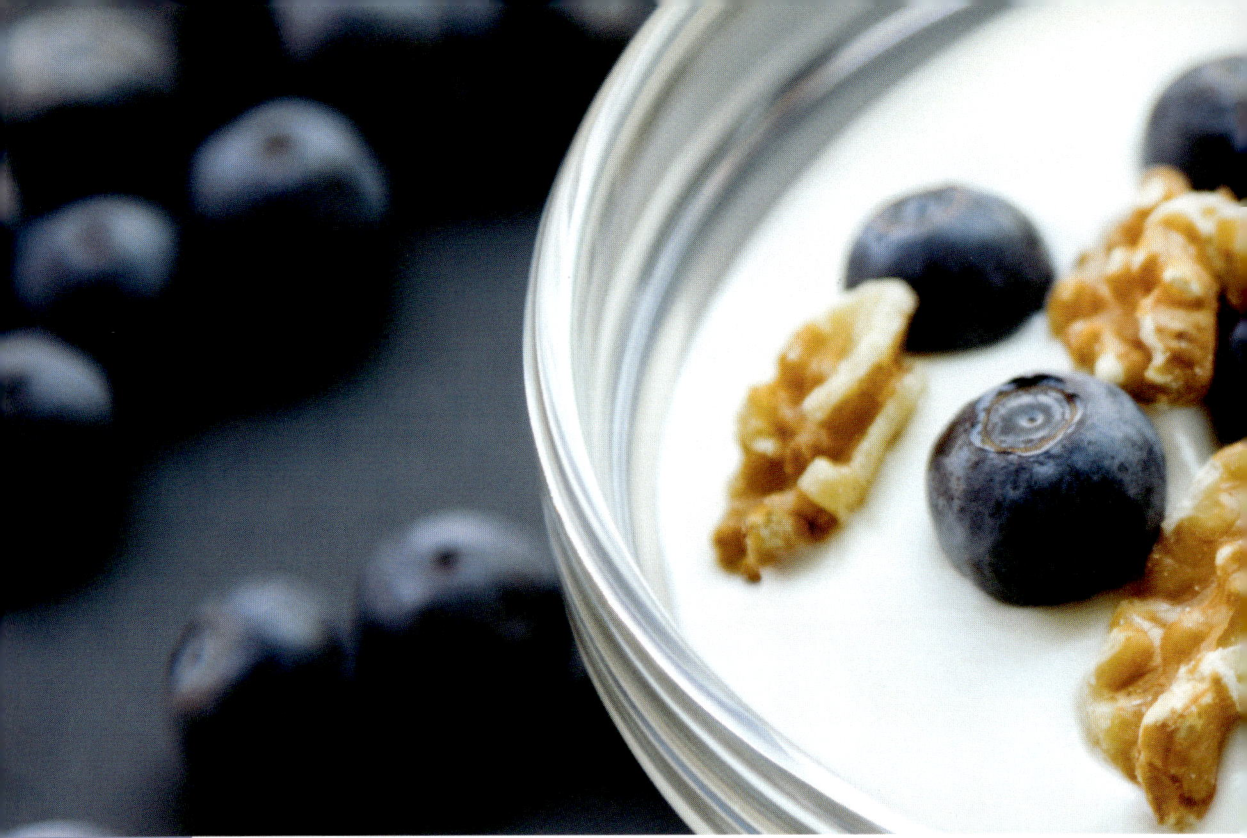

Fruit and yoghurt

SERVES
1

A quick grab and go yoghurt bowl snack.

Ingredients

½ cup plain yoghurt

½–1 cup of berries or fresh fruit

Optional 10 nuts for flavour and crunch.

To save money, buy yoghurt in bulk and portion it into containers as needed.

You can add your fruit and have this ready to grab from the fridge.

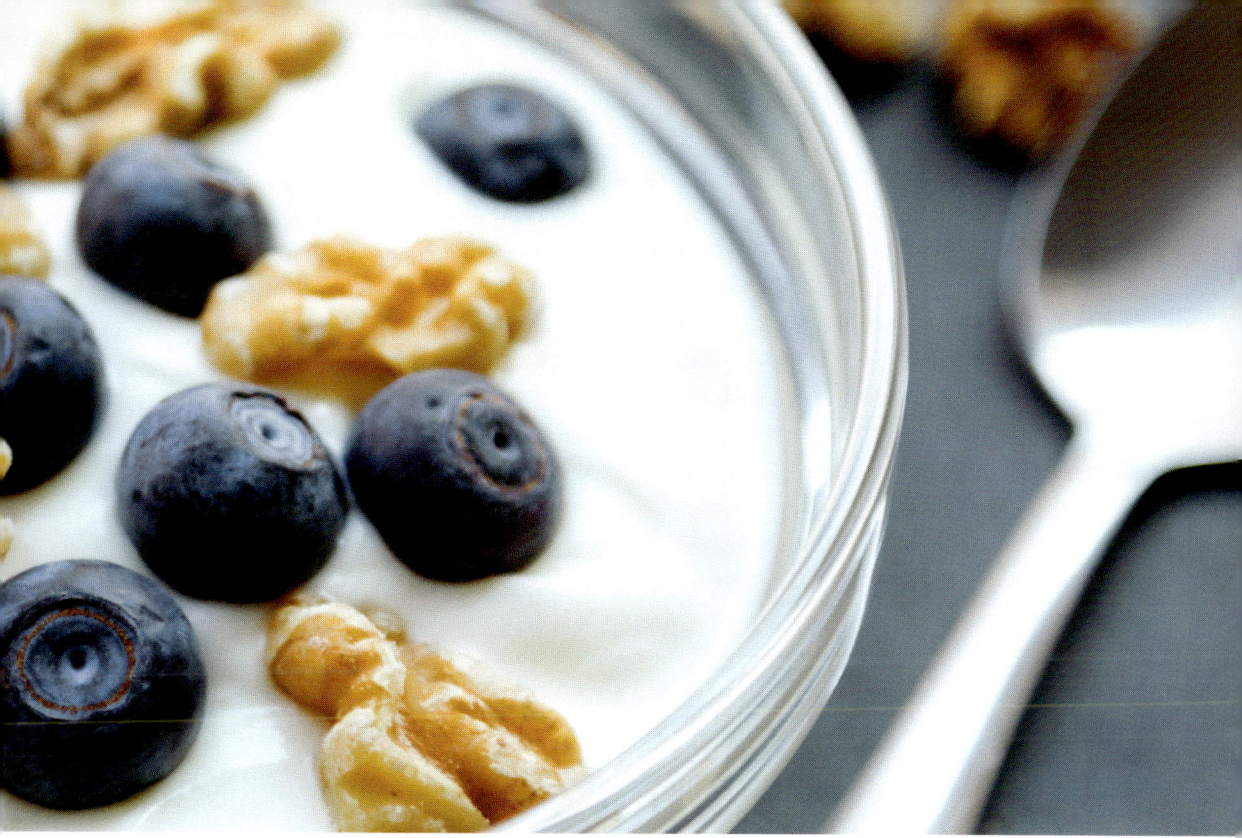

Method

1. Place approx ½ cup plain yoghurt in a bowl
2. Top with a ½–1 cup berries or fruit of choice
3. Garnish options: 3 tablespoons chopped nuts and seeds or home made muesli or granola (see page 66 and 68).

Greek, natural or unflavoured yoghurt is a healthier choice.

Add your own fruit for flavour and some nuts and seeds for crunch!

Bliss balls
Chocolate

MAKES
20

A very simple high fibre snack that can have the kids involved too!

Ingredients

2½ cups dates soaked in enough water just to cover the dates

2 cups almond meal

½ cup cacao

½ cup shredded coconut

Desiccated coconut for coating

Method

1. After soaking dates for 2 hours blend with the water* in food processor for 20-30 seconds
2. Add cacao, coconut and almond meal and blend for a further 20 seconds
3. Mix, roll and coat in desiccated coconut
4. Keep in fridge or freezer.
5. Keep in freezer.

**Note: too much water used in this step will cause a very wet mixture. If unsure, drain all the water and reserve to add back in for desired consistency in step 3.*

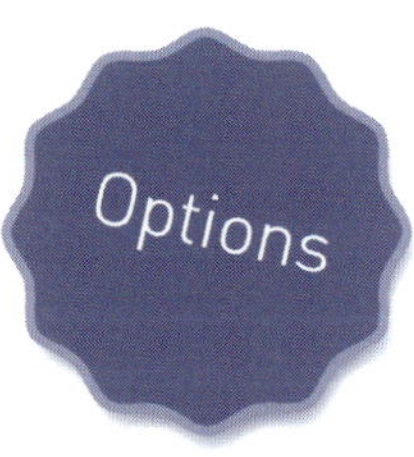

Dust in cacao powder, crushed nuts or sesame seeds.

SNACKS

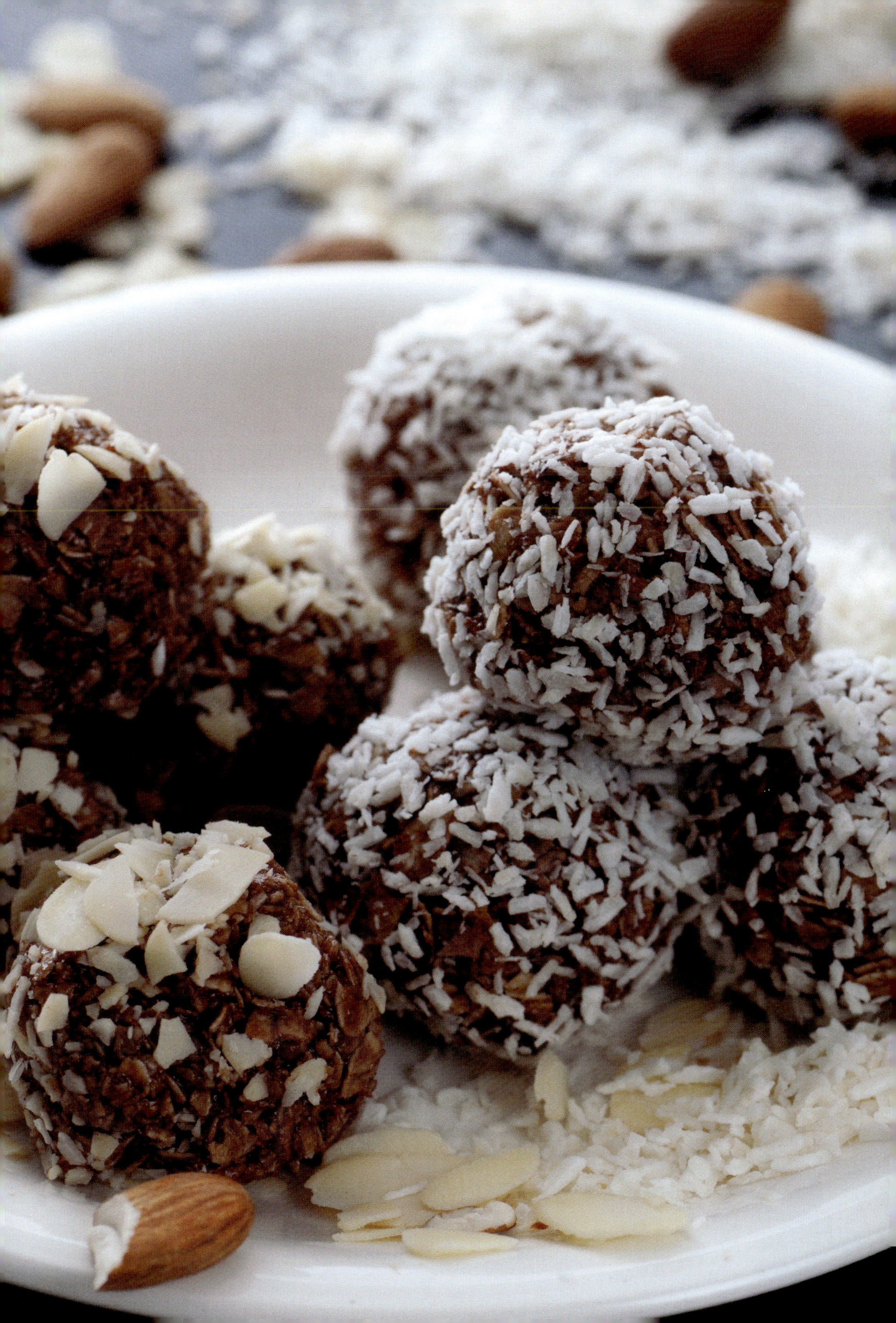

Bliss balls
Peanut butter

MAKES
12

Ingredients

120g pitted dates

1 cup almond meal

½ cup shredded/ desiccated coconut plus extra for coating

150g crunchy or smooth natural peanut butter

2-3 tablespoons water to mix

Method

1. Add dates, meal and coconut to form a crumb in the blender
2. Place the crumb in a bowl. Add peanut butter and some water to mix
3. Roll and coat in desiccated coconut
4. Store in fridge or freezer.

Bliss balls
Lemon cashew

MAKES
20

Ingredients

500g cashews

2 lemons and zest of one lemon

Desiccated coconut for coating

Method

1. Put cashews in blender to create crumb consistency
2. Transfer to a bowl. Add lemon juice and zest
3. Leave to rest for 30-60 minutes to form thick consistency
4. Roll and coat in desiccated coconut. Store in fridge or freezer.

Bliss balls
Nut free chocolate

MAKES
12

Ingredients

120g pitted dates (soaked)

1 cup shredded coconut

½ cup cacao

1 cup oats

¼ cup water

Desiccated coconut, Milo or sprinkles for rolling

Method

1. Combine dates (with water), oats, shredded coconut and cacao in blender until it forms a crumb-like consistency
2. Transfer mixture to bowl and add water as needed to form a dough
3. Roll and coat with desiccated coconut (or Milo/ sprinkles for a treat)
4. Store in fridge and allow to set for a few hours.

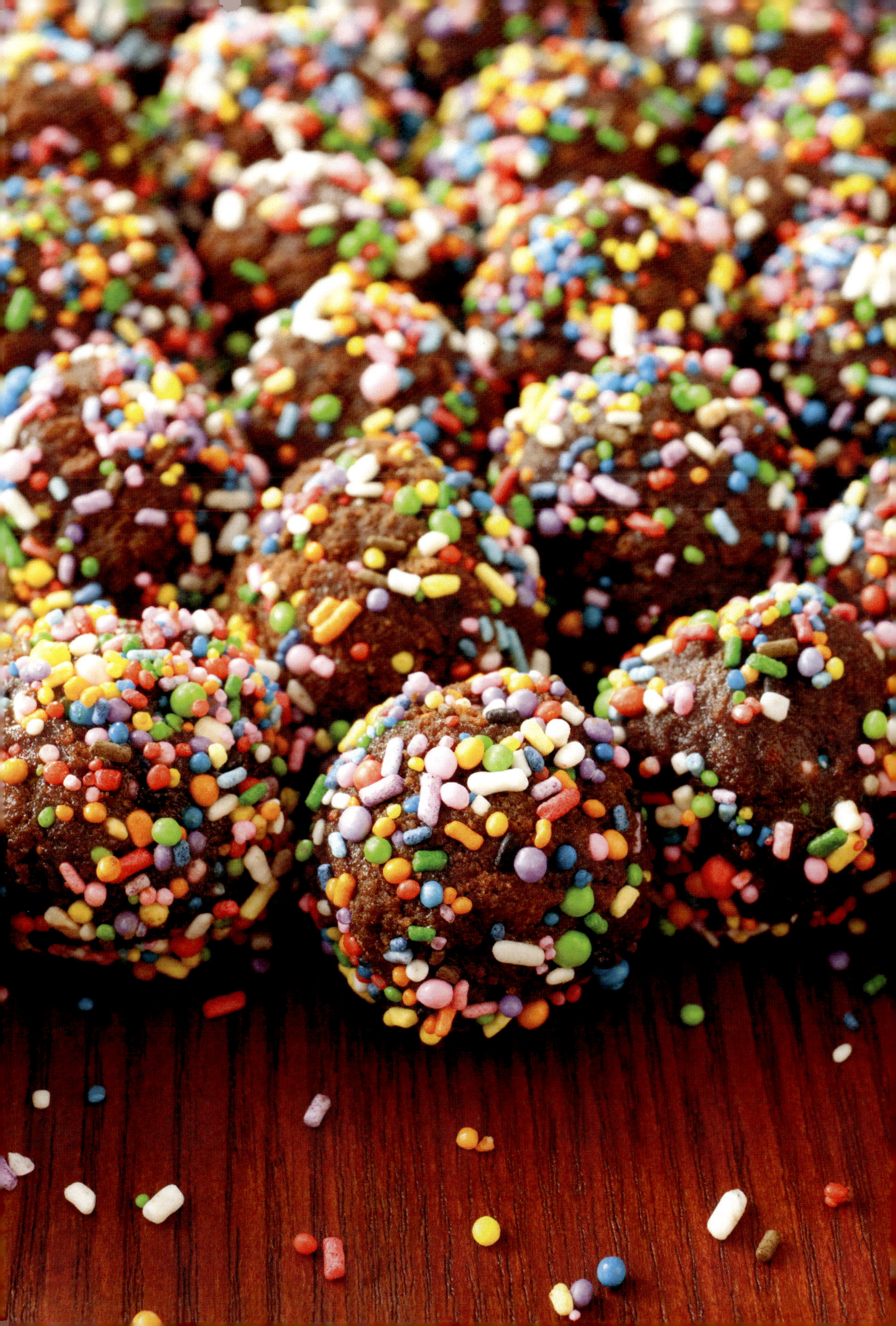

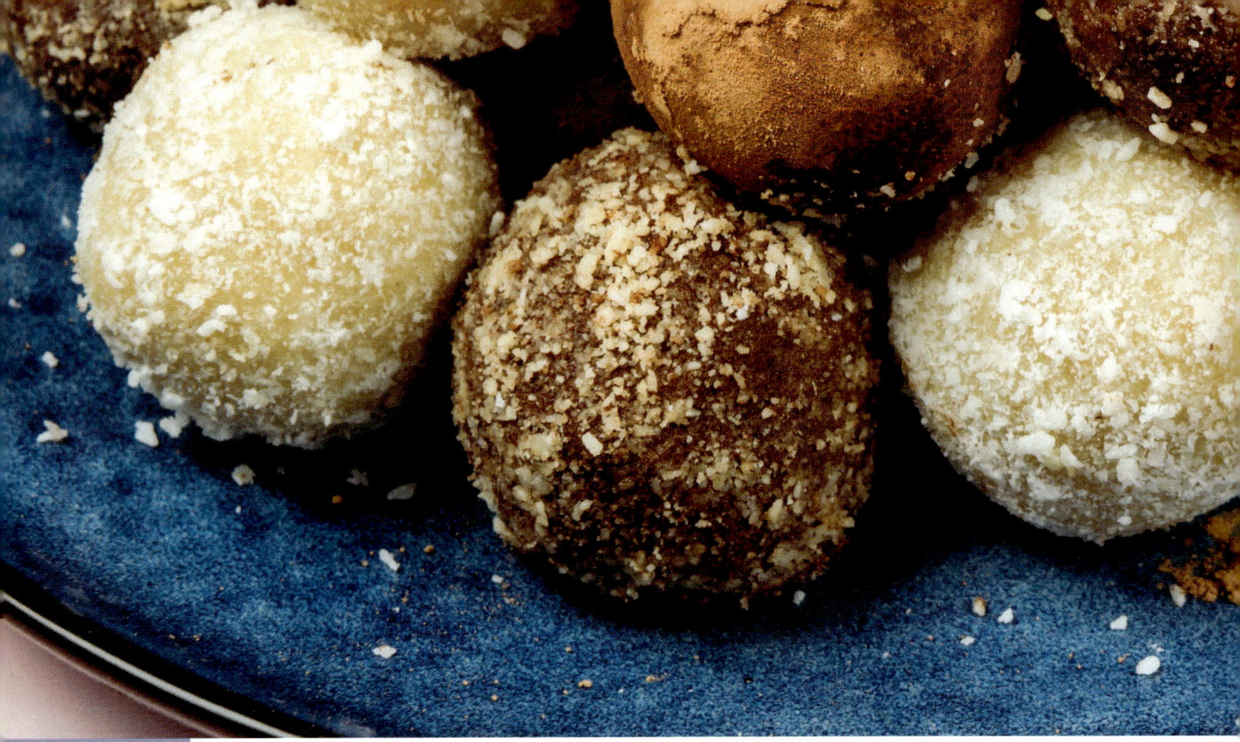

Bliss balls
Carrot and pecan

MAKES
20

Ingredients

½ large carrot, grated

1 cup pecans

1 cup oats

1 cup pitted dates soaked in warm water (enough to cover the dates)

1 cup shredded coconut

1 teaspoon of ground cinnamon

1 cup blended pecans/ walnuts or desiccated coconut for rolling

Method

1. Grate carrot
2. Place pecans, carrot, oats, dates (with water), cinnamon and shredded coconut in blender and blend until mixture combines
3. Roll and coat in coconut or nuts
4. Refrigerate for 2 hours or overnight to set.

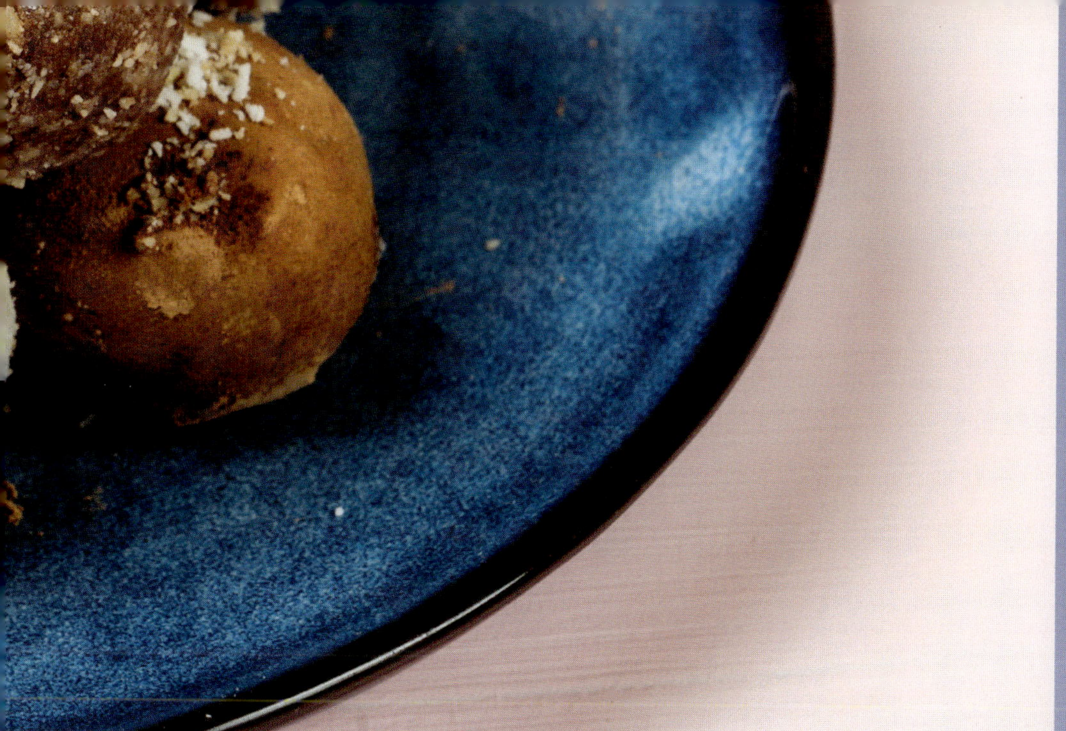

Carrot balls
No nuts

MAKES
20

Great for lunch boxes.

Ingredients

1 large carrot, grated

1 cup oats

1 cup dates covered in warm water

1 cup shredded coconut

1 teaspoon ground cinnamon – adding more to taste

Method

1. Follow instructions above, leaving out any nuts
2. Coat in coconut. Store in fridge or freezer.

Chocolate muffins

MAKES
18-24

Ingredients

2 large bananas mashed

4 eggs

¾ cup olive oil

¾ cup milk (or alternative – almond or coconut)

1-2 tablespoons honey (optional – still delicious without but include if you would like it sweeter/for the kids)

3 cups almond meal

½ cup cacao powder

¾ cup shredded coconut

¾ teaspoon baking soda (bicarb)

1 teaspoon gluten-free baking powder

Method

1. Preheat oven to 160°C
2. Mash banana in large bowl and combine with eggs, olive oil, milk and honey
3. Add almond meal, cacao, coconut, baking soda and baking powder
4. Put into silicone or lined muffin pans (¾ full)
5. Bake for 20-25 minutes. (Check by lightly pressing top. If it springs back they are ready)
6. Store in fridge up to 3 days or freeze up to a month.

Tip

Occasionally add some dark chocolate chips to step 3 or scatter over the top before baking.

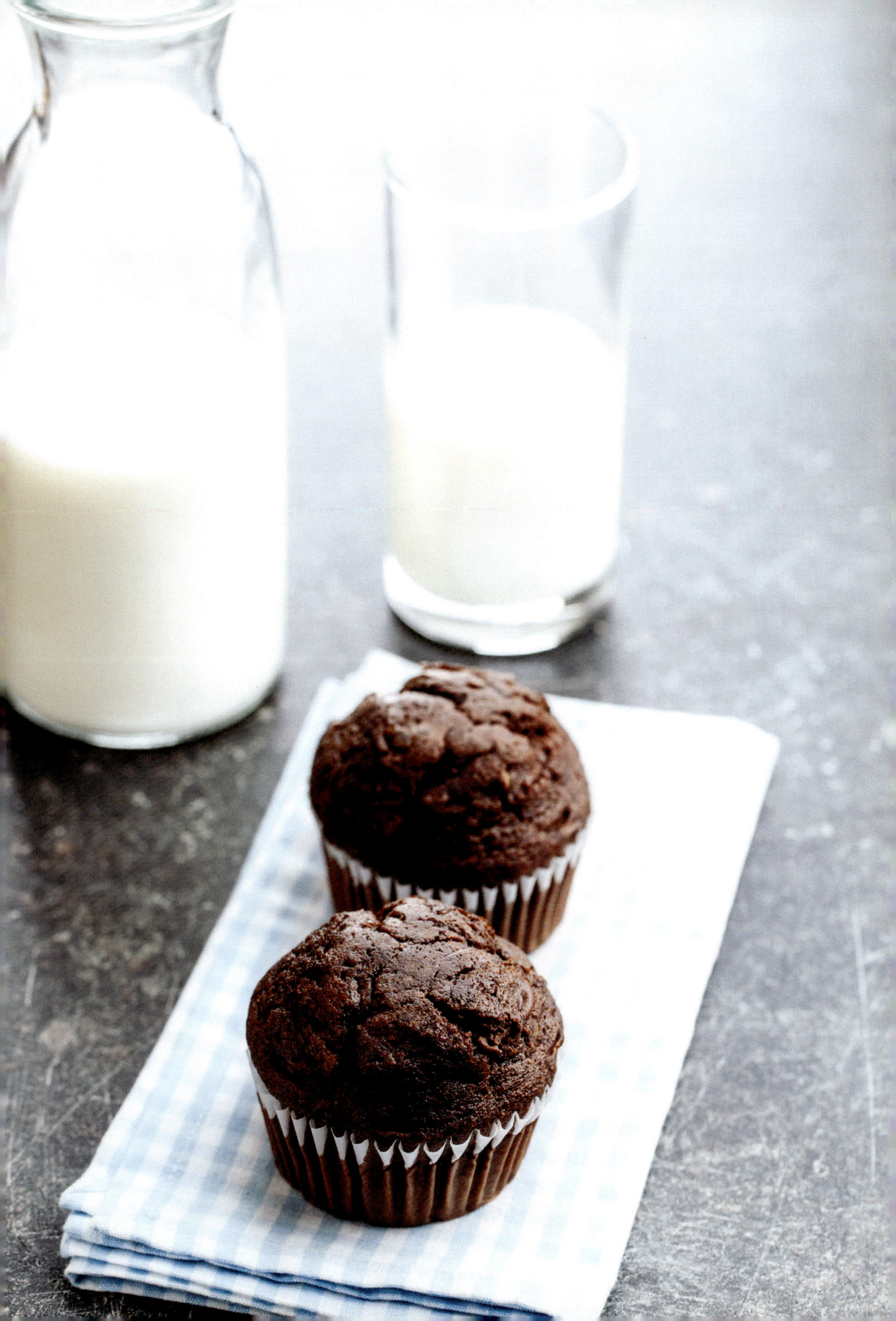

Signature muffins

Blueberry, walnut or banana

MAKES
10-12

Ingredients

2 cups almond meal

¾ cup chopped walnuts or 1 punnet of blueberries

2 tablespoons flaxseeds

1 generous tablespoon ground cinnamon

2 teaspoons baking powder

2 large eggs

1 cup apple sauce (or extra mashed banana)

¼ cup olive oil

¼ cup plain yoghurt

2 mashed bananas (add 1 extra mashed banana for banana muffins)

Method

1. Mix dry ingredients. Add wet ingredients and bananas
2. Stir ingredients together well
3. Place in muffin tins that are well greased or lined
4. Bake at 170°C for about 45 minutes until well cooked/dark.

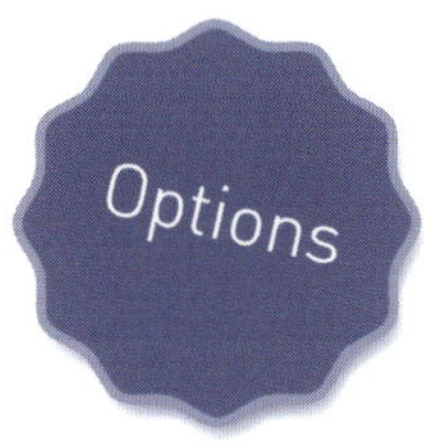

You can eliminate blueberries and walnuts and instead add a few dark choc chips to the top of the mixture once in muffin tins.

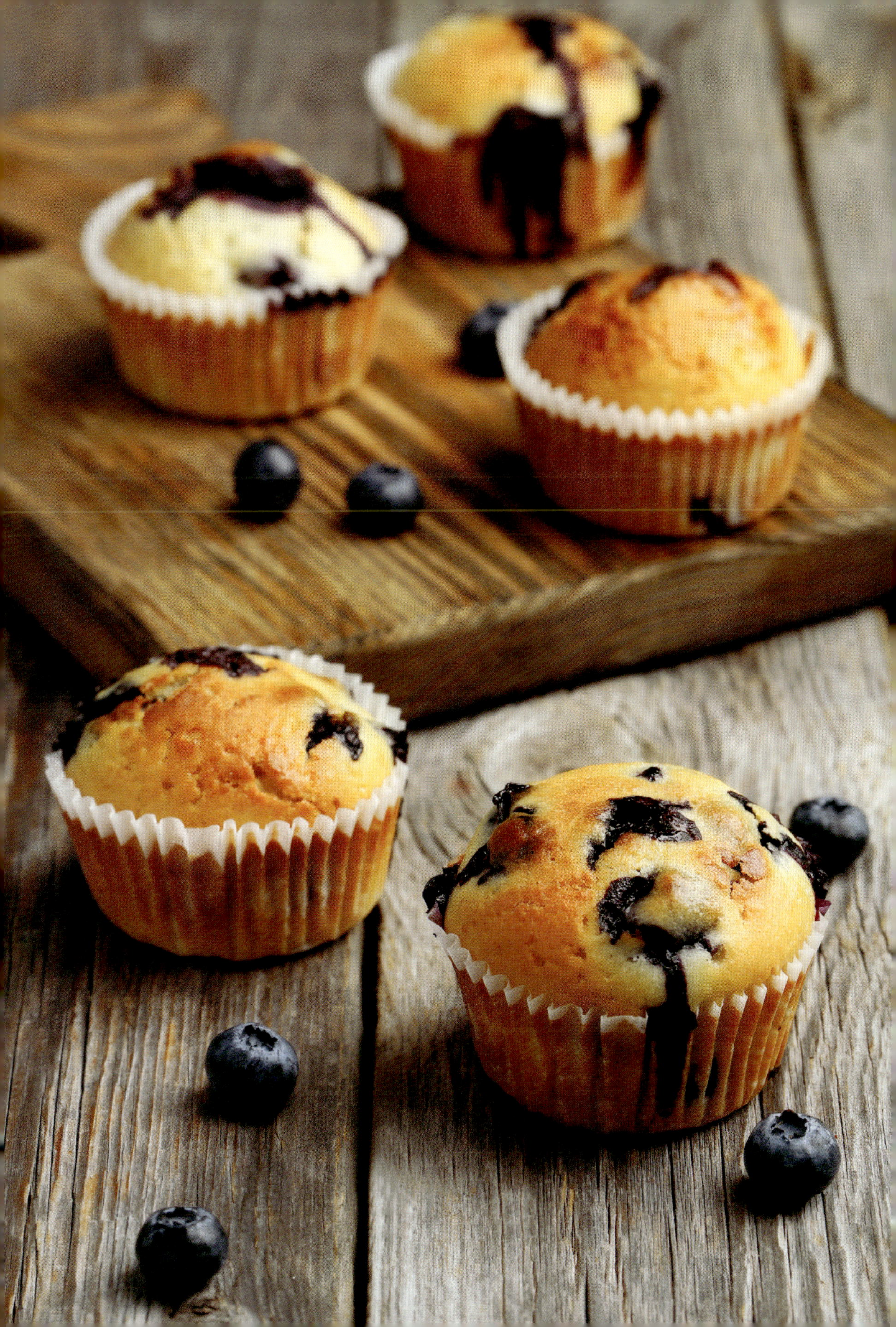

Banana Bread

SERVES
10

Toasted this makes a great breakfast with fresh banana and a drizzle of honey or scoop of fresh yoghurt.

Ingredients

4 mashed bananas

1½ teaspoons baking powder

¼ teaspoon sea salt

3 eggs

¼ cup olive oil

½ teaspoon cinnamon

1½ teaspoons vanilla essence

2 cups almond meal

½ cup rolled oats (this can be replaced with an extra ½ cup almond meal)

¼ cup pepita seeds (topping)

1 sliced banana (topping)

Method

1. Combine mashed banana, baking powder, salt, eggs, oil, cinnamon and vanilla into a bowl and mix well
2. Add the almond meal and oats and mix through lightly. It's important not to over-mix so just until it's combined
3. Line a loaf tin with baking paper at the base and the sides
4. Spoon mixture into the loaf tin. Sprinkle additional cinnamon, banana circles and pepitas on top
5. Bake for 45 minutes or until skewer inserted comes out clean
6. Remove from the oven and allow to cool completely before removing from the tin.

Store in the fridge once cooled or cut and wrap up in single serving sizes and freeze.

Variation: instead of pepitas top with banana circles and choc chips for the kids.

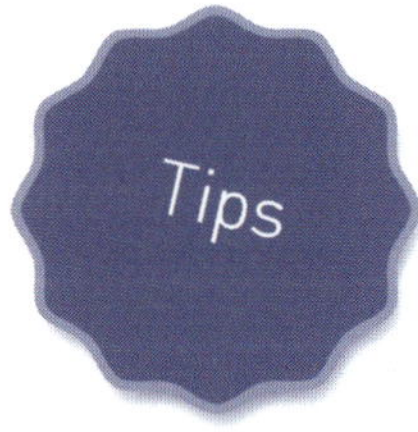

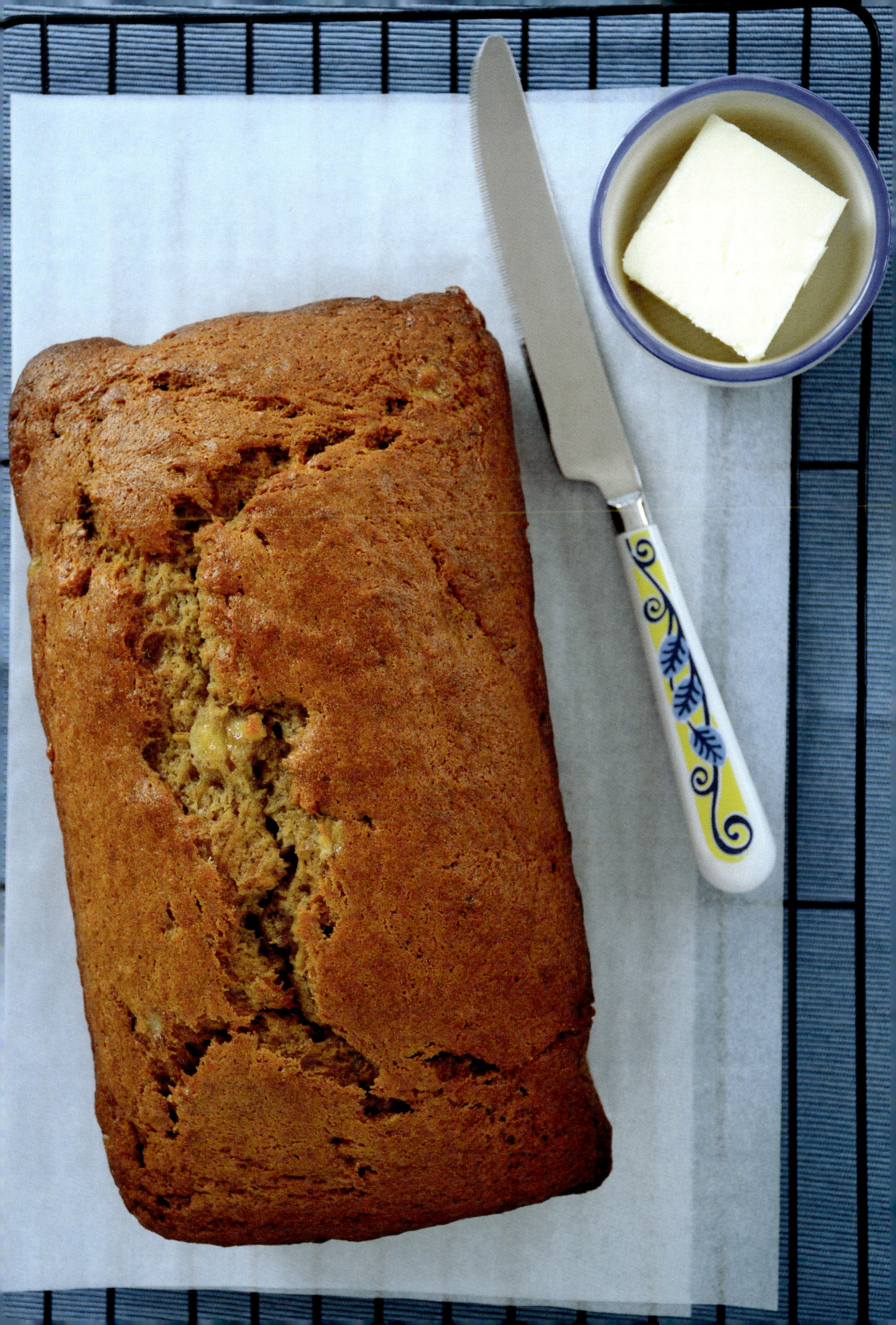

Oat and seed muesli bar

SERVES
10

Ingredients

1 cup rolled oats

¼ cup pepitas

¼ cup sunflower seeds

2 tablespoons sultanas, goji berries or chocolate chips (or you can leave this out)

¾ cup shredded coconut

1/3 tablespoon coconut oil

1/3 cup honey

1 teaspoon vanilla extract

1 teaspoon cinnamon

Method

1. Preheat oven to 160°C
2. Line tray with baking paper and set aside
3. Mix oats, pepitas, sunflower seeds and coconut in a bowl and set aside
4. On stove top or in microwave, add coconut oil, honey and vanilla and bring to the boil, then remove from the heat
5. Combine both mixtures and mix until well combined
6. Press firmly into a 20cm x 20cm tin. For crunchy bars follow steps 7-9. For chewy bars place as is in the refrigerator to set for a few hours. Cut into bars and store in the fridge.
7. Bake for 15 minutes or until starting to turn golden brown.
8. Remove from oven and allow to cool COMPLETELY on tray then refrigerate overnight before cutting. This allows them to set.
9. Cut into 10 bars and store in an airtight container.

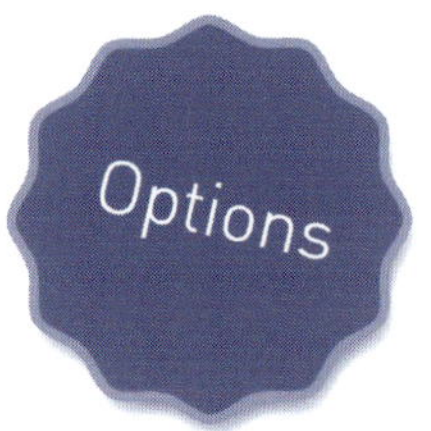

Add chopped nuts and or goji berries instead of sultanas.

Gluten-free /nut lovers' version – replace oats with 1 cup almond meal and 1 cup coconut, add 1 cup chopped almonds/walnuts, ¼ cup each of pepitas/sunflower seeds. Add 2 tablespoons of almond spread to wet mixture as listed above.

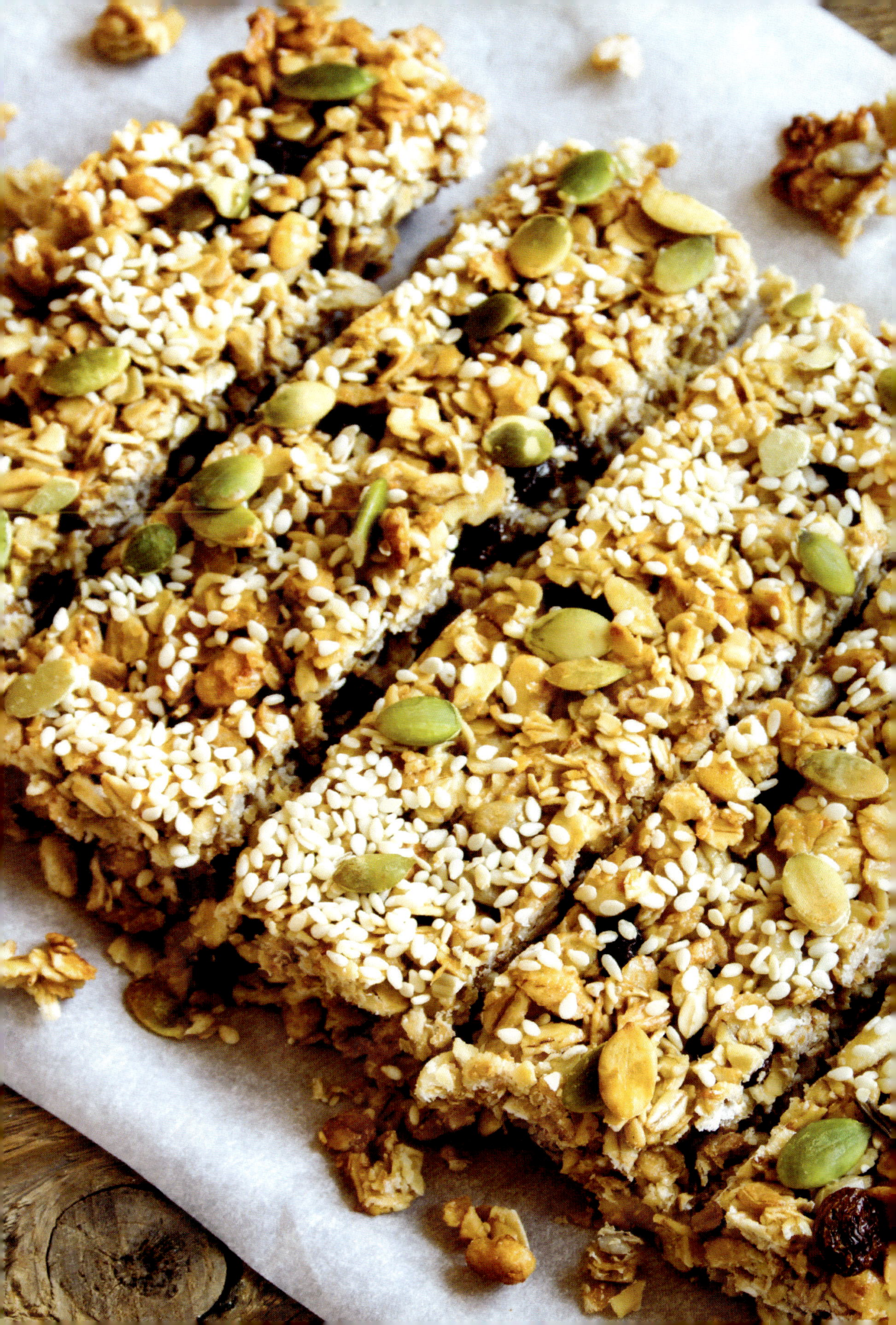

Brownies

MAKES
8-10

Ingredients

1 cup pitted dates

1 cup roasted macadamias

½ cup desiccated coconut

1 tsp vanilla bean paste

2 tablespoons raw cacao

Method

1. Line tin with baking paper
2. Place all ingredients in food processor bowl and process for at least 30 seconds until it comes together
3. Press mixture into tin and flatten
4. Refrigerate for 4 hours.

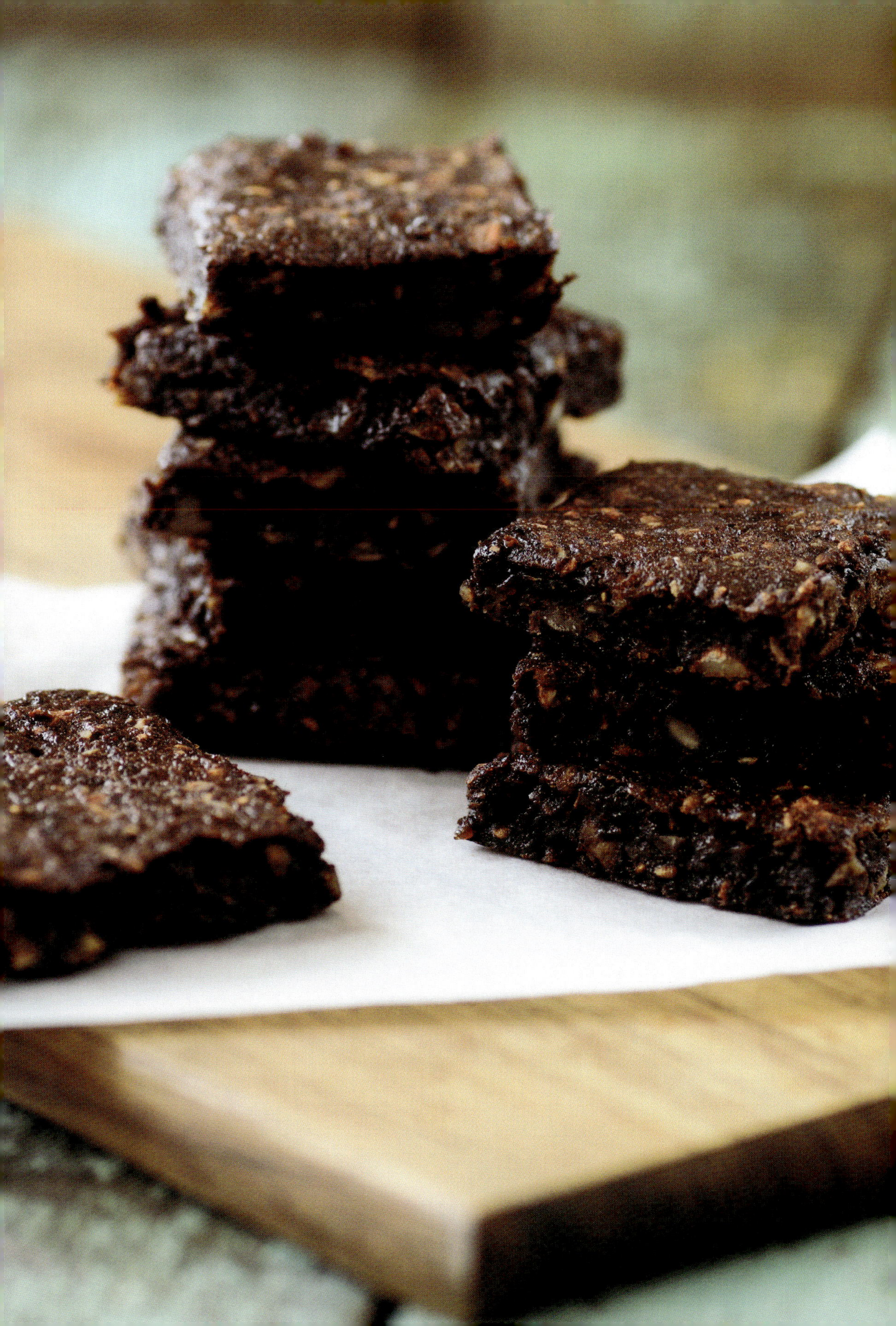

Wrap

SERVES
1

Wraps can often be a lighter alternative to the classic sandwich.

Try mountain bread or a grain wrap.

Gluten free wraps are available – See Foodfix4life App for recommendations.

Ingredients

1 mountain bread wrap

avocado

3 salmon slices – you could also use drained tin tuna or shredded chicken

Chopped tomato

Spinach leaves

Lime

Method

1. Mash avocado, tuna and chopped tomato
2. Add a squeeze of lime and pepper
3. Spread onto wrap over spinach leaves
4. Roll.

Kids get bored with sandwiches all the time.

Try a wrap, rice paper rolls or salad as a lunch alternative.

LUNCH / DINNER

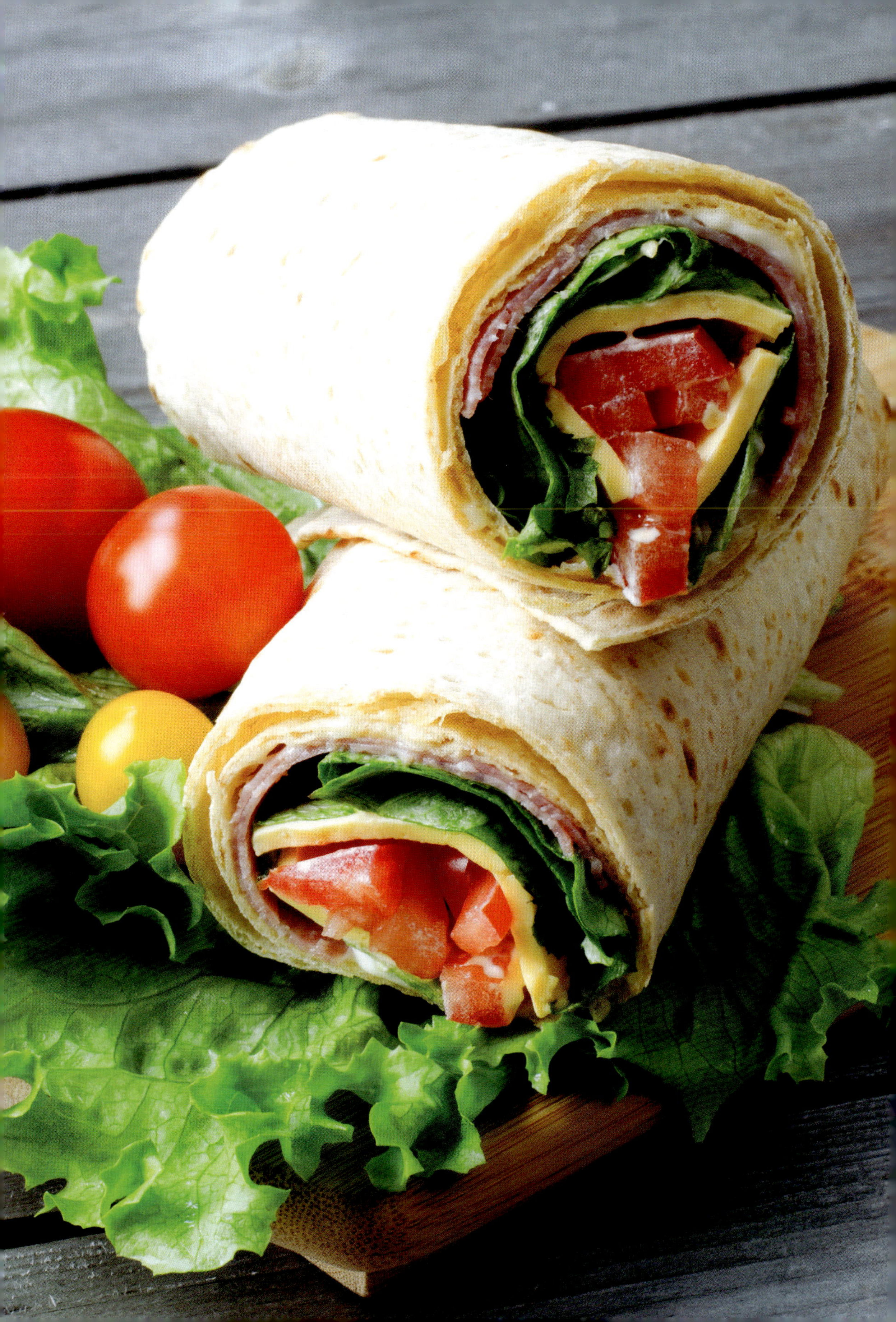

Rice paper rolls

MAKES
12

Ingredients

12 x 22cm round rice papers

1 cucumber, cut into thin strips

1 red capsicum, cut into thin strips

1 large carrot, cut into thin strips

1 small avocado, cut into thin slices

50g snow pea sprouts, ends trimmed

¾ cup coriander leaves

Soy sauce

Juice of one lime

1 teaspoon of honey

Method

1. Soak one rice paper roll in a bowl of warm water for a few seconds until soft
2. Mix the soy sauce, honey and lime juice together
3. Put a few slices of each vegetable on the rice paper leaving about 3 cm at each end
4. Fold in each end of the rice paper. Then roll the paper up to make the veggie roll
5. Dip the rolls into the sauce for a scrumptious lunch.

Use any leftover ingredients or add a protein such as chicken or salmon.

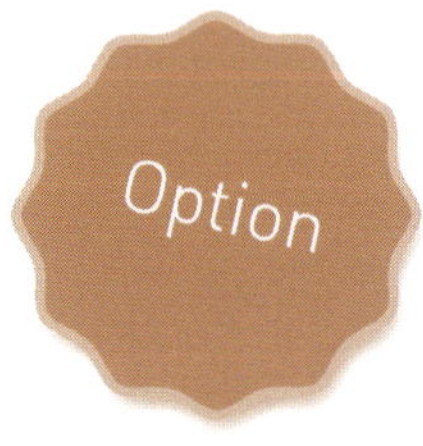

LUNCH / DINNER

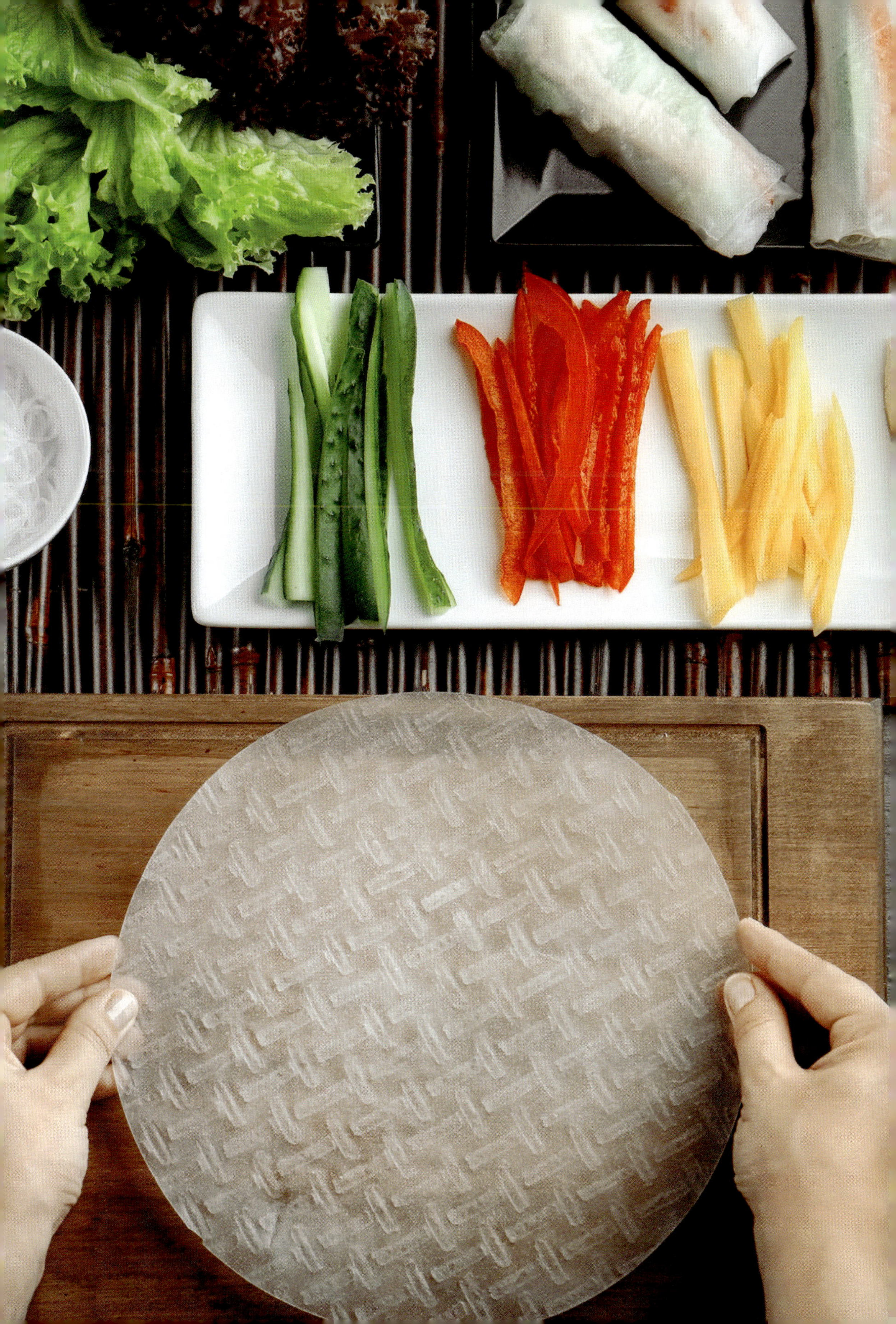

Sweet potato, spinach & fetta pie

SERVES
8

Ingredients

1 large sweet potato

400g kale and spinach. (e.g. 1x 280g bag of baby spinach plus 140g bag pre-cut kale)

200g fetta

8 eggs whisked

½ teaspoon nutmeg

Flaked almonds

Olive oil (extra virgin) or butter for cooking

Additional seasonings of choice (garlic, chilli etc)

Method

1. Slice sweet potato thinly (½cm) and place on bottom and sides of pie dish to cover entirely
2. Sauté spinach and kale in olive oil or butter (additional garlic or chilli etc if you wish)
3. When cooked place in pie dish on top of sweet potato
4. Top with crumbled fetta (or other cheese)
5. Whisk eggs and nutmeg, pour into dish over the spinach and fetta
6. Top with flaked almonds, to cover the pie entirely
7. Bake about 40 minutes until cooked.

Pumpkin salad

SERVES
1

Ingredients

120g baked or steamed pumpkin

Raw veggies diced plus baby spinach

Balsamic vinegar/glaze

30g crumbled fetta

6 walnuts

Add protein: 120-150g grilled chicken

Method

1. Place spinach on platter
2. Add pumpkin and any vegetables such as semi sun dried tomato's.
3. Place walnuts and fetta cubes followed by a drizzle of balsamic.

Baked potato with toppings

SERVES 1

Ingredients

1 medium to large white or sweet potato

Protein of choice such as ham/bacon/salmon

Veggies of choice such as tomato, corn or leftovers such as broccoli

Grated tasty cheese/ crumbled fetta

Method

1. Bake potato in oven until cooked
2. Slice and remove some of the flesh for stuffing/topping
3. In a bowl, mix the flesh, ham, tomato and corn and place as stuffing in the potato
4. Top with grated cheese and re-bake for 10 minutes (until cheese has melted).

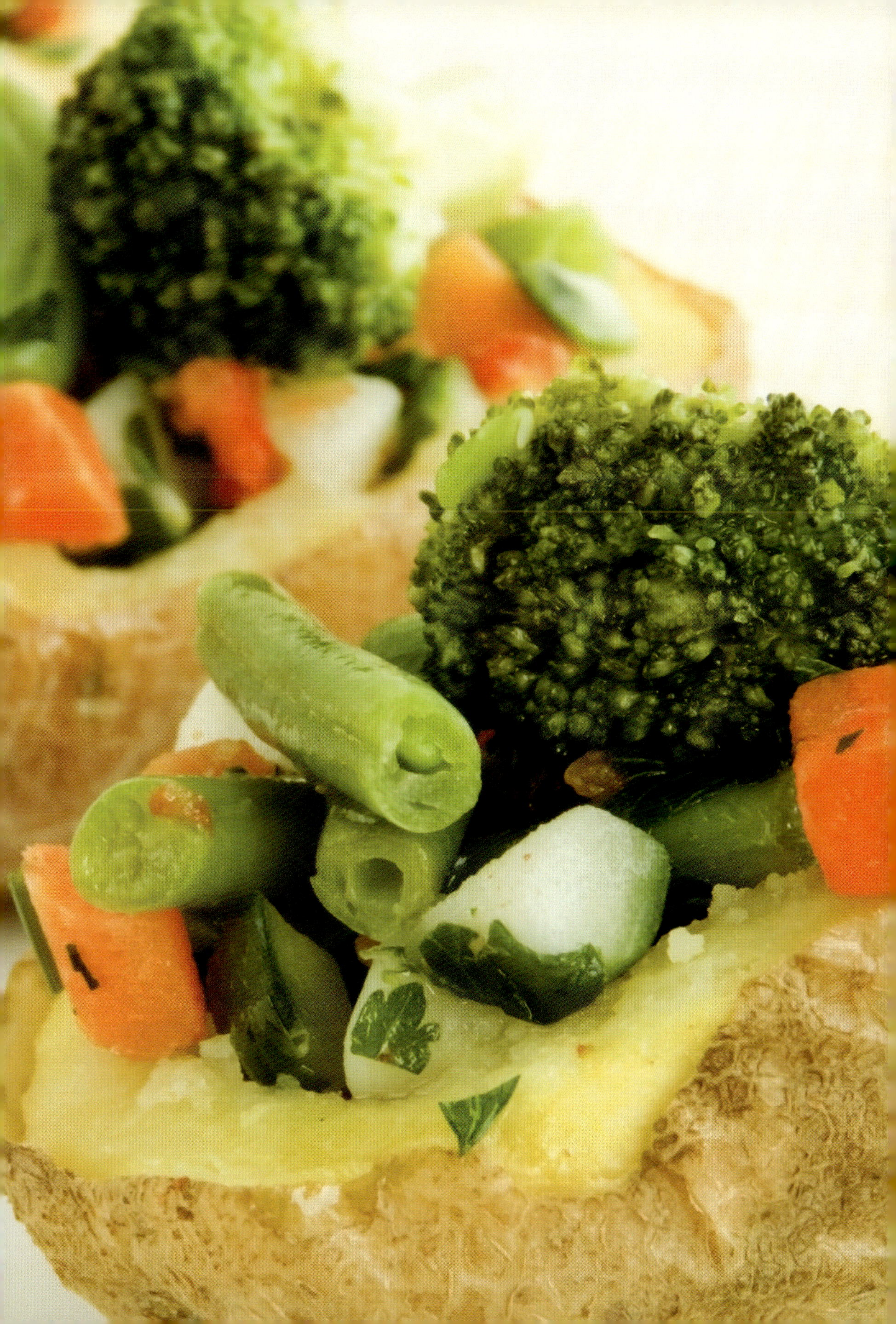

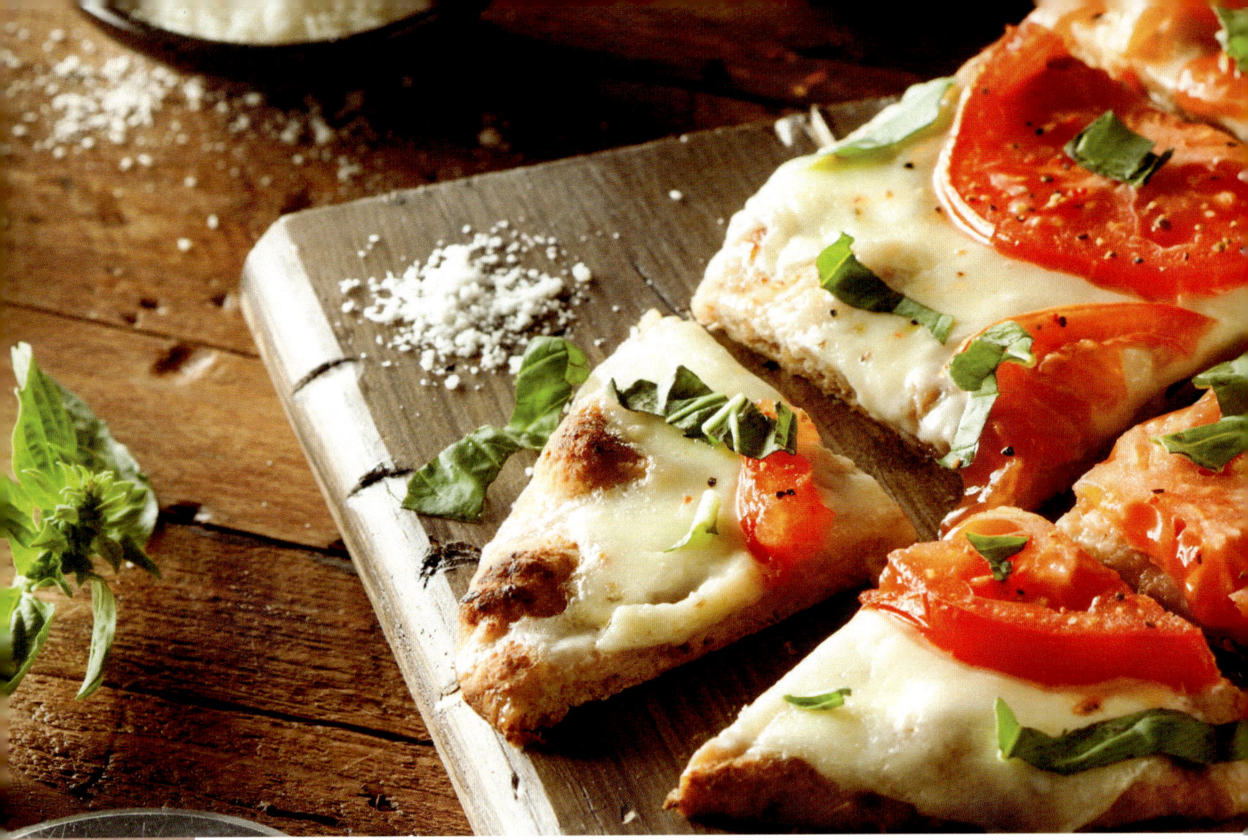

Mini pizzas

SERVES
1

A great meal that gets the kids involved too.

You can easily do homemade pizza bases using flours of choice such as gluten free.

Use ingredients that kids will like such as quality shaved ham, grated cheese and pineapple.

A mix of tasty and mozzarella cheese for the kids works well.

LUNCH / DINNER

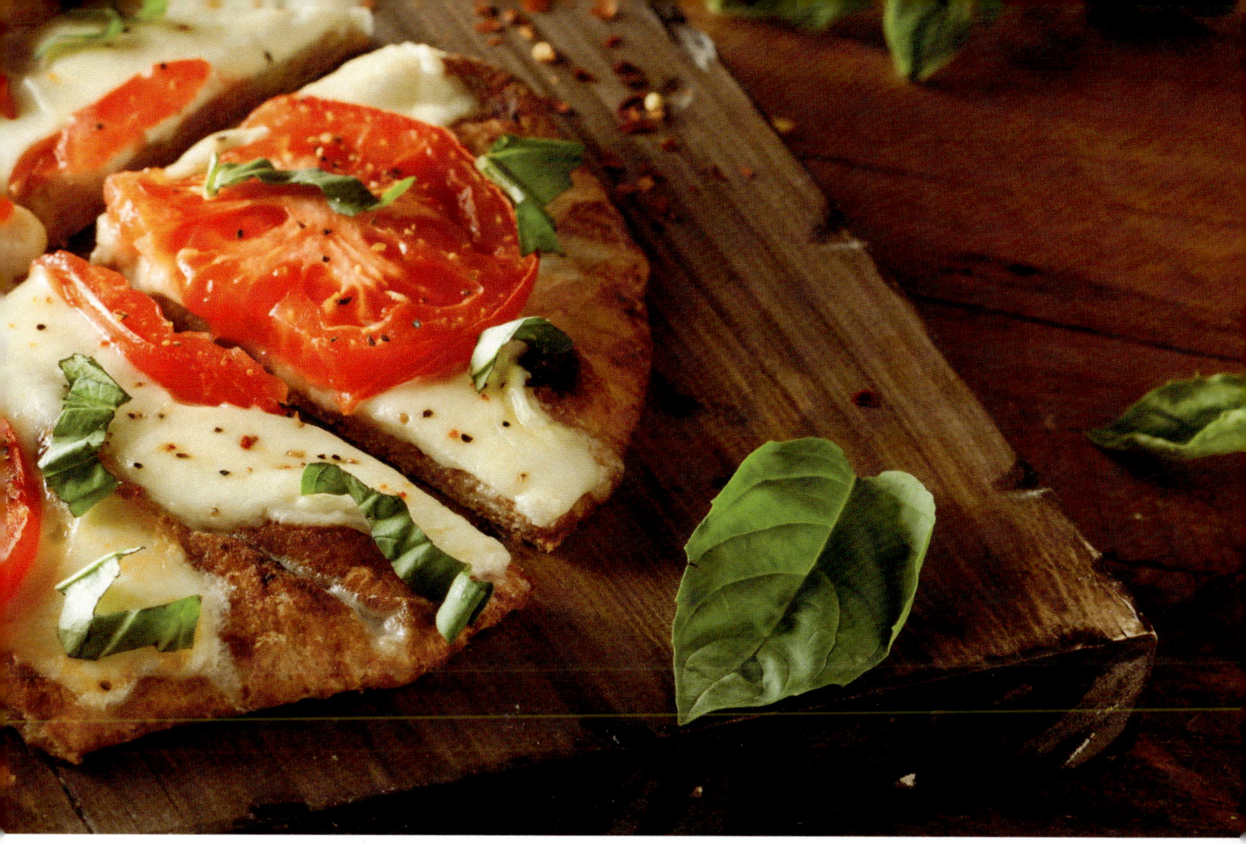

Ingredients

Wholemeal/grain pitta bread (or your choice of base)

Tomato paste

Mixed Italian herbs

Fresh basil

Mushrooms

Olives

Shredded chicken/quality shaved ham

50g fetta / ½ cup grated mozzarella

Method

1. Spoon a few tablespoons of tomato paste into a bowl and mix in herbs and chopped basil
2. Spread over pitta base
3. Top with chicken, mushroom, olive and fetta/mozzarella
4. Bake in preheated oven on 160°C for 10-15 minutes.

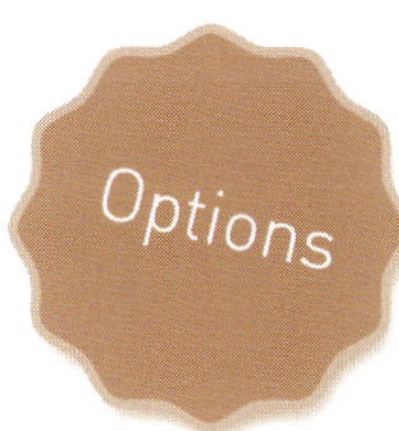

Pumpkin, broccoli, sundried tomato, spinach and fetta

Chicken, pumpkin and fetta

Ham and cheese

Olives, sun-dried tomatoes, eggplant, red capsicum, onion, mushroom

Base options – an English muffin, slice of toasted bread, bought or homemade pizza base, low-carb base e.g. low carb pizza base mixes-found online at www.lovepbco.com or at health food stores.

Tuna and potato balls

MAKES
10-15

Ingredients

1 large can of tuna, drained

1 cup cooked mashed potato

½ onion fried in olive oil

2 eggs

1 teaspoon cumin

Salt (black pepper, chilli or paprika optional)

1 teaspoon lemon juice

1 cup breadcrumbs

Olive oil for cooking

Method

1. Mix the tuna, potato, 1 of the eggs, onion, lemon, salt and spices in a mixing bowl until all the ingredients are combined. Taste and adjust seasoning

2. Whisk the remaining egg with a fork. Place the breadcrumbs in a bowl. Form balls with a teaspoon of the tuna mixture. Dip in the egg and then coat in breadcrumbs. Place in the fridge for 10 minutes.

3. Heat the oil then fry the balls for a couple of minutes and place on paper towel to drain. Serve with dipping sauce.

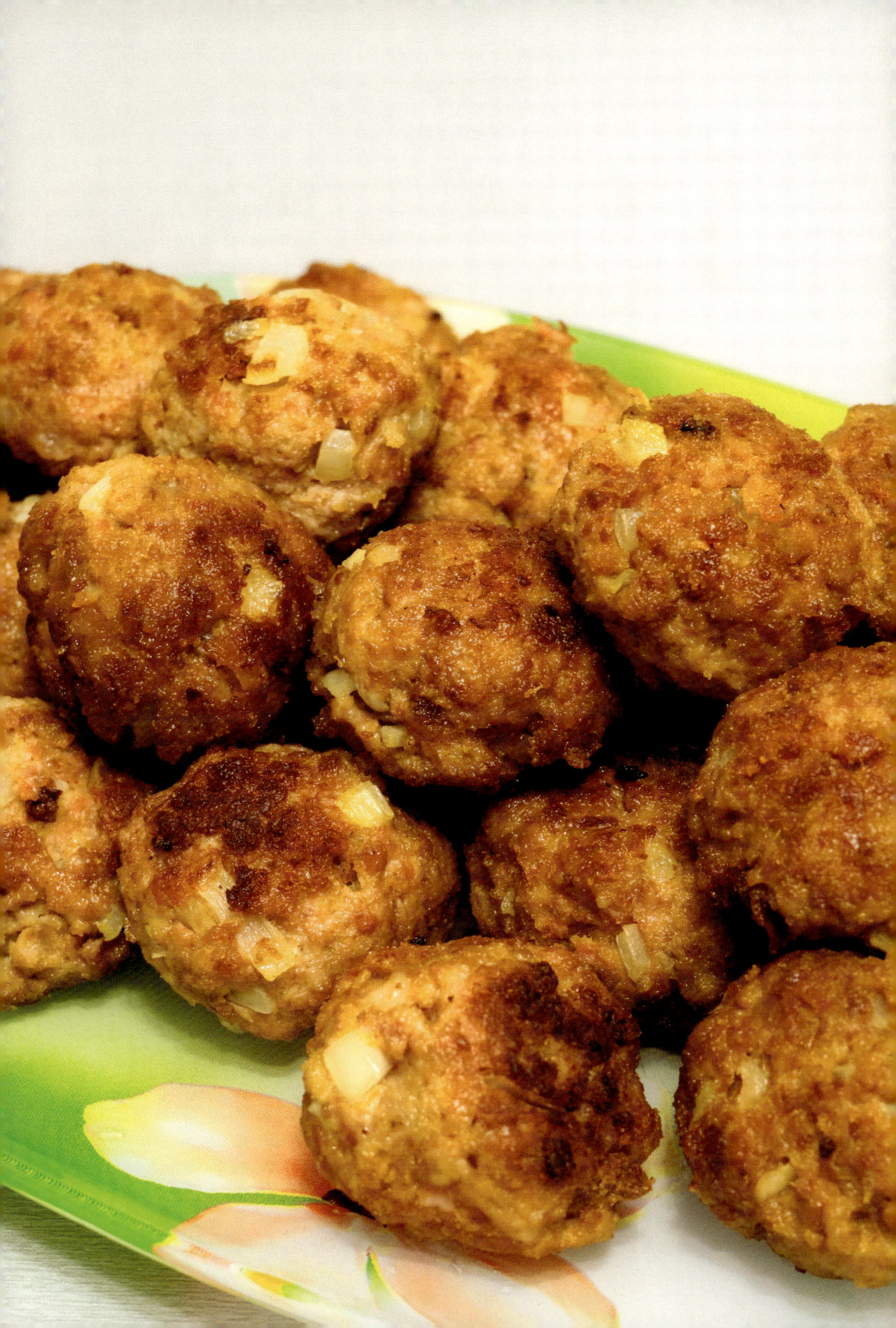

Burger and chips

MAKES
1

Homemade is always best!

Patty could be made of beef, lentil, chicken or fish.

Ingredients

Bun of choice (for those wanting less carb try using a grilled large mushroom as the bun)

Cheese

Lettuce

Tomato

Avocado

Potato/sweet potato cut into wedges

Choice of sauce – tomato, barbecue, mayonnaise, chilli, mustard

Beef patty ingredients:

- 200g mince of your choice
- 1 tbsp chopped parsley
- ¼ cup grated parmesan
- ¼ cup breadcrumbs
- 1 egg
- salt and pepper

Method

1. Mix together patty ingredients and shape to form 2 patties, grill/bake. Set aside. These can be made the day before.
2. Drizzle chip wedges with olive oil and place chips on baking paper in oven on 180°C for about 1 hour until cooked
3. Make your masterpiece ... Bun + avo and chilli + lettuce + tomato + cheese + chicken patty + a side of chips!

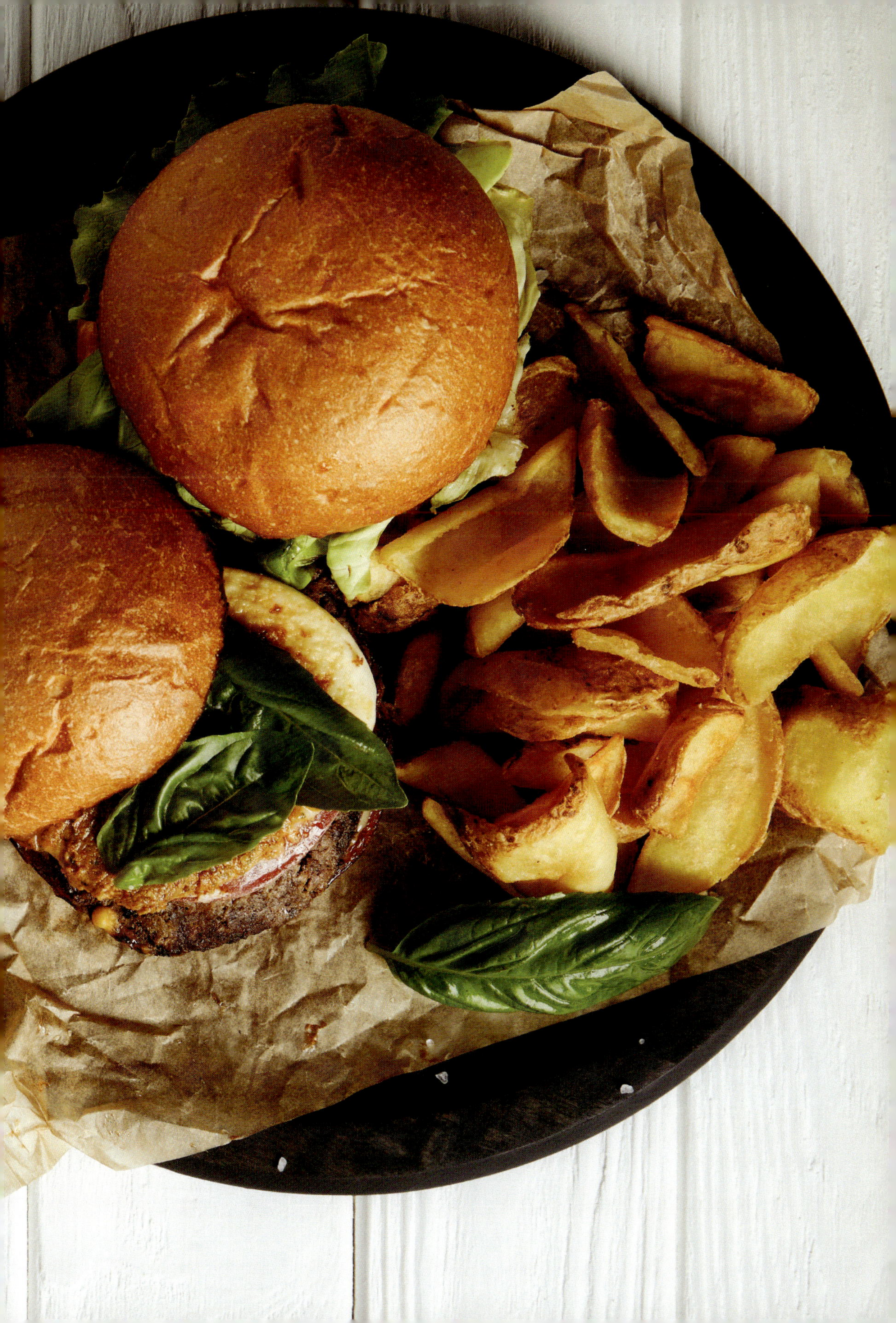

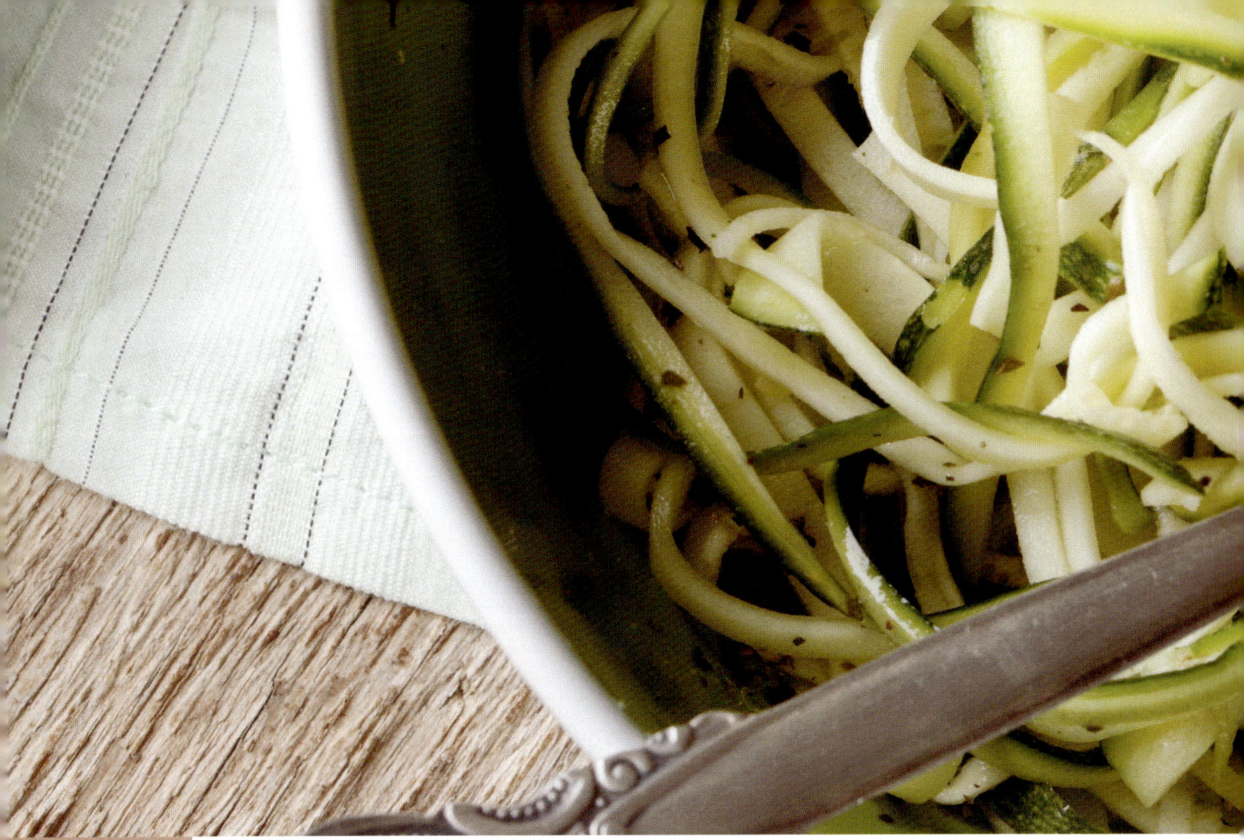

Spaghetti

A favourite staple for most families

LUNCH / DINNER

Options

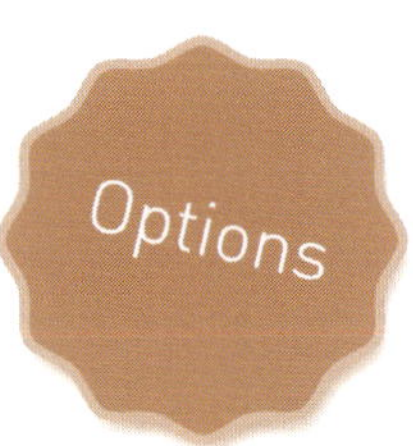

For those who are gluten free please choose gluten free pasta varieties

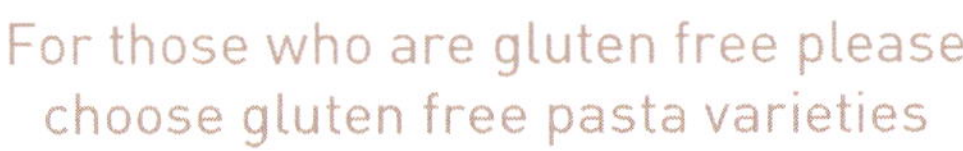

You can also try sweet potato noodles/ carrot noodles which are readily available at the supermarket

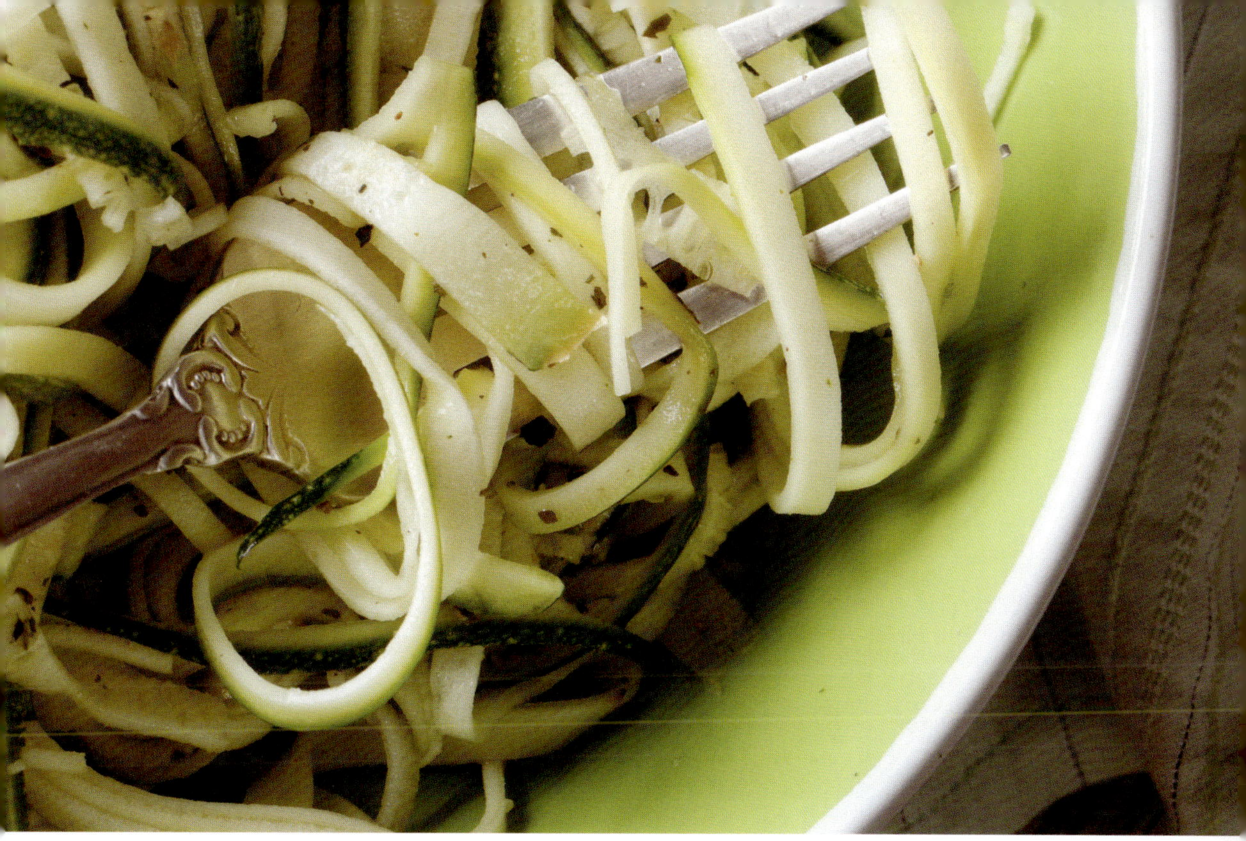

Ingredients

Thin spaghetti or shaped pasta such as penne or trivelle

Pasta sauce, either bottled or homemade

Grated parmesan cheese

Method

1 Cook pasta and drain

2 Add sauce and stir through

3 Add grated parmesan cheese.

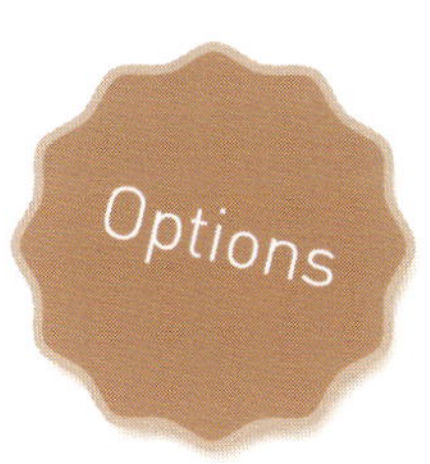

Low carb options are:

Slendier pasta found in the health food section of your supermarket

Zucchini noodles found in the produce section at the supermarket ready to add the sauce.

Quick homemade pasta sauce

SERVES
4

Ingredients

2 x 400g tin chopped peeled tomatoes

2 tablespoons tomato paste

1 clove crushed garlic

½ onion diced

Optional: grated carrot and zucchini and/or finely chopped mushrooms

¼ cup herbs such as basil and oregano

¼ teaspoon nutmeg

1tablespoon olive oil

1 teaspoon sugar (optional)

Salt, pepper to season

Method

1. Heat oil and add the onion and garlic and stir for a few minutes
2. Add tomato paste and stir through
3. Add the tomatoes, stir and reduce heat until thickens slightly
4. Add sugar, salt, pepper, basil, oregano and season as required.

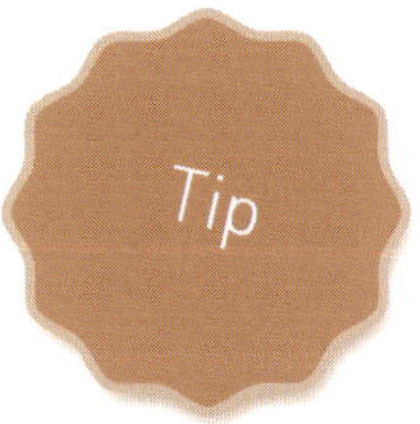

Pasta sauce is a great way to hide some veggies for the kids.

Don't tell them and they won't know the difference! I always top the pasta with some grated parmesan.

That helps hide any green bits!

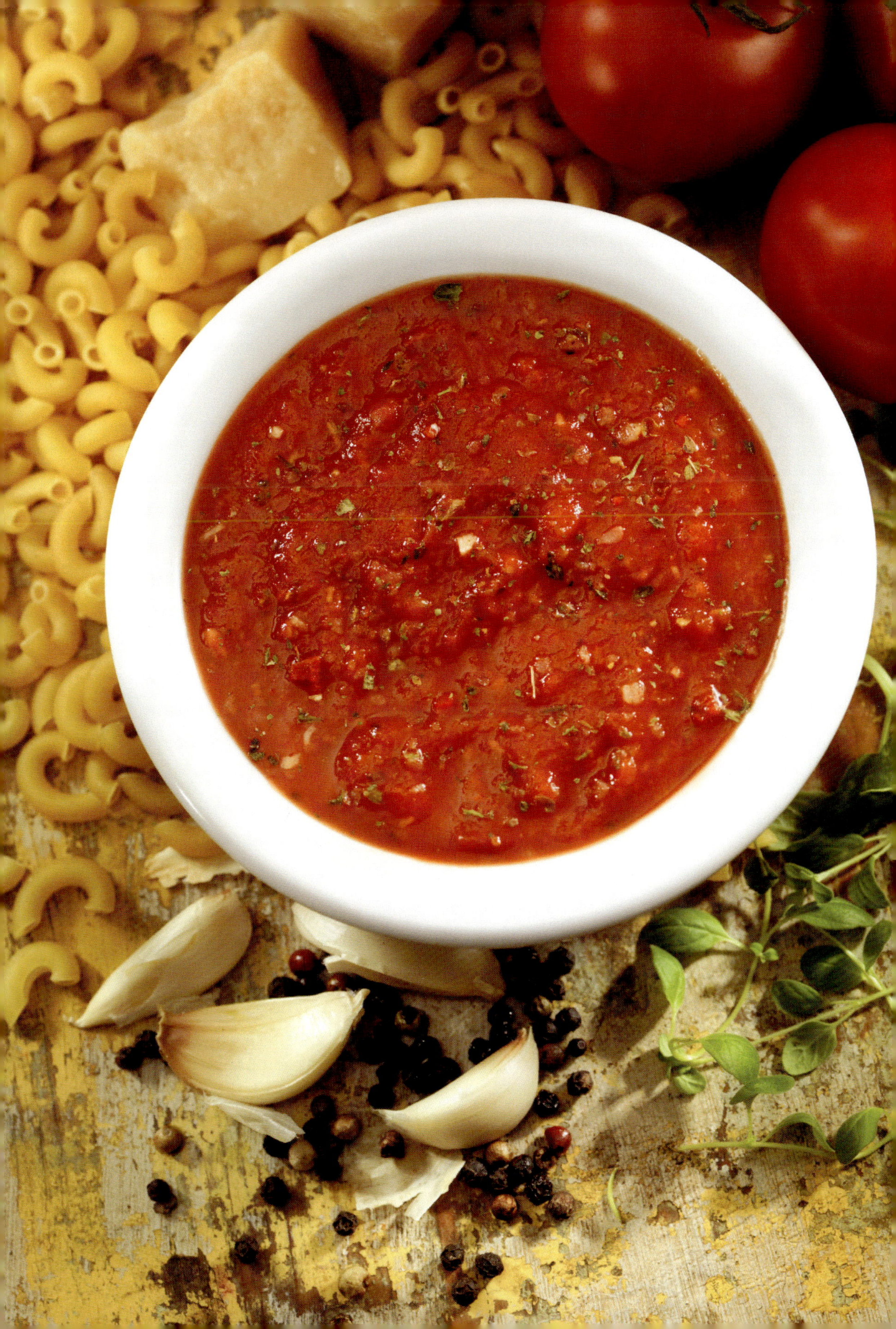

Crumbed chicken pieces/nuggets

SERVES
4

This is a weekly staple in many households.

It can be baked or fried and the leftovers (if there are any) are delicious the next day.

Ingredients

4 chicken breasts cut into thin slices

Eggs whisked for coating

Parsley (optional)

Parmesan

Breadcrumbs (option to use quinoa or gluten free crumbs)

Method

1. Place chicken breast in bowl with beaten egg
2. Chop 2 tablespoons parsley and add to a bowl with breadcrumbs
3. Add ½ cup finely grated parmesan to the breadcrumbs and stir to combine
4. Remove a piece of chicken, one at a time and coat in the breadcrumb mixture. Press firmly.
5. Place chicken on baking paper to bake in oven or place in hot pan with olive oil to pan fry.

Oven – spray the top of the chicken with olive oil spray then bake for about 25 minutes or until cooked, turning once.

Pan fry – make sure oil is hot before starting. These require just a few minutes on each side. Place on paper towel before serving.

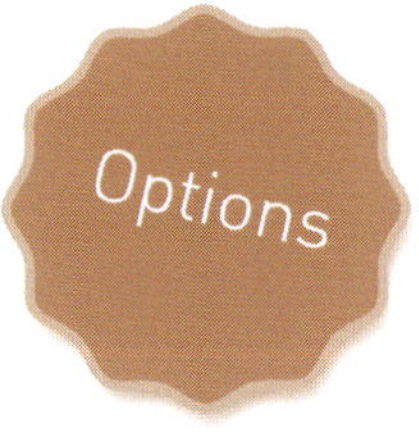

Use thin slices of veal, fish fillets, prawns or thicker chicken cubes for nuggets.

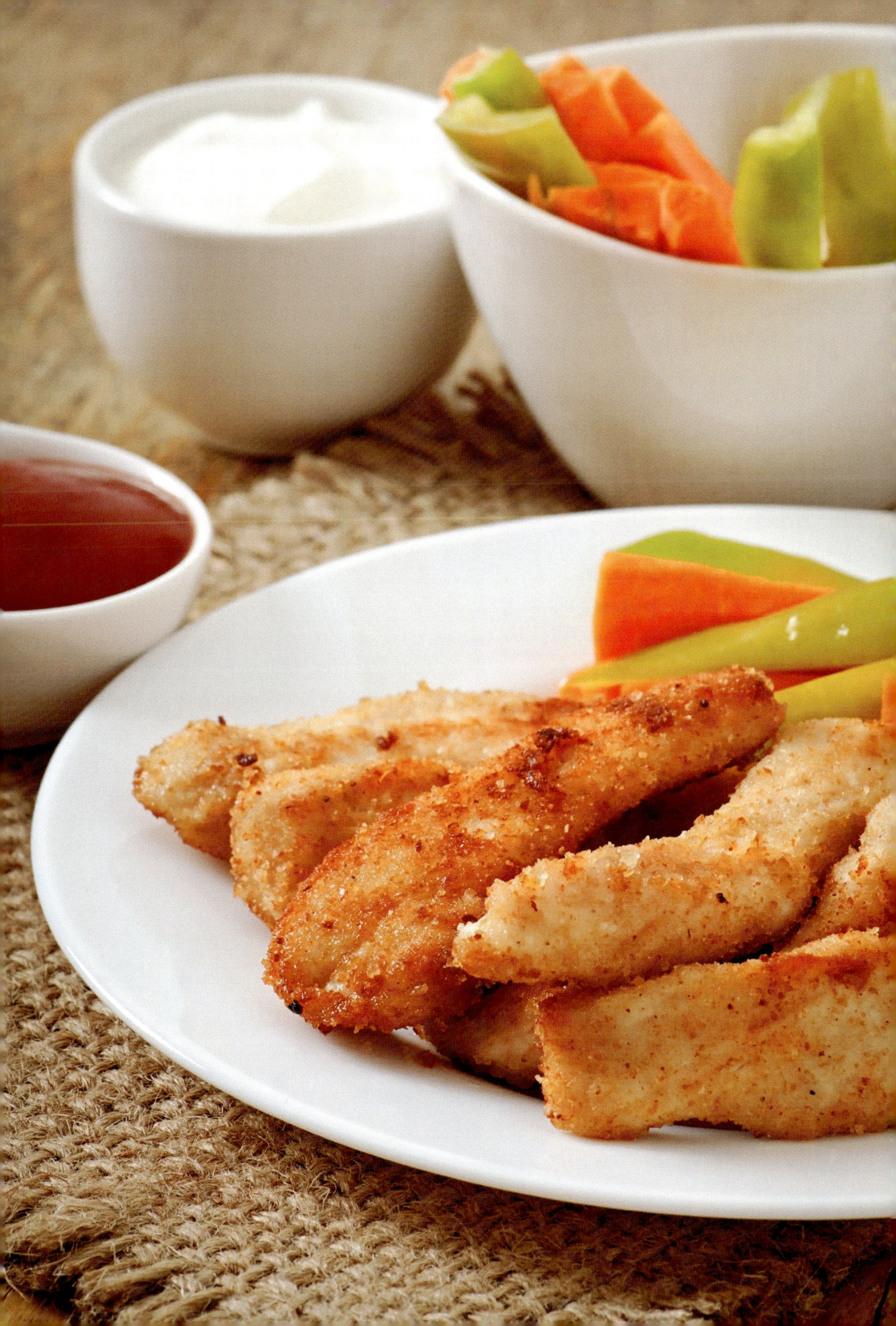

Grilled seafood plate

SERVES
2

This is where you pick your favourite seafood for the barbecue.

Ingredients

2 fish fillets

4 Baby octopus

4 Calamari

4 Prawns

4 Scallops

Method

1. Marinate in extra virgin olive oil and herbs or spices of choice
2. Grill on hot barbecue plate until cooked
3. Serve hot with a side Greek salad.

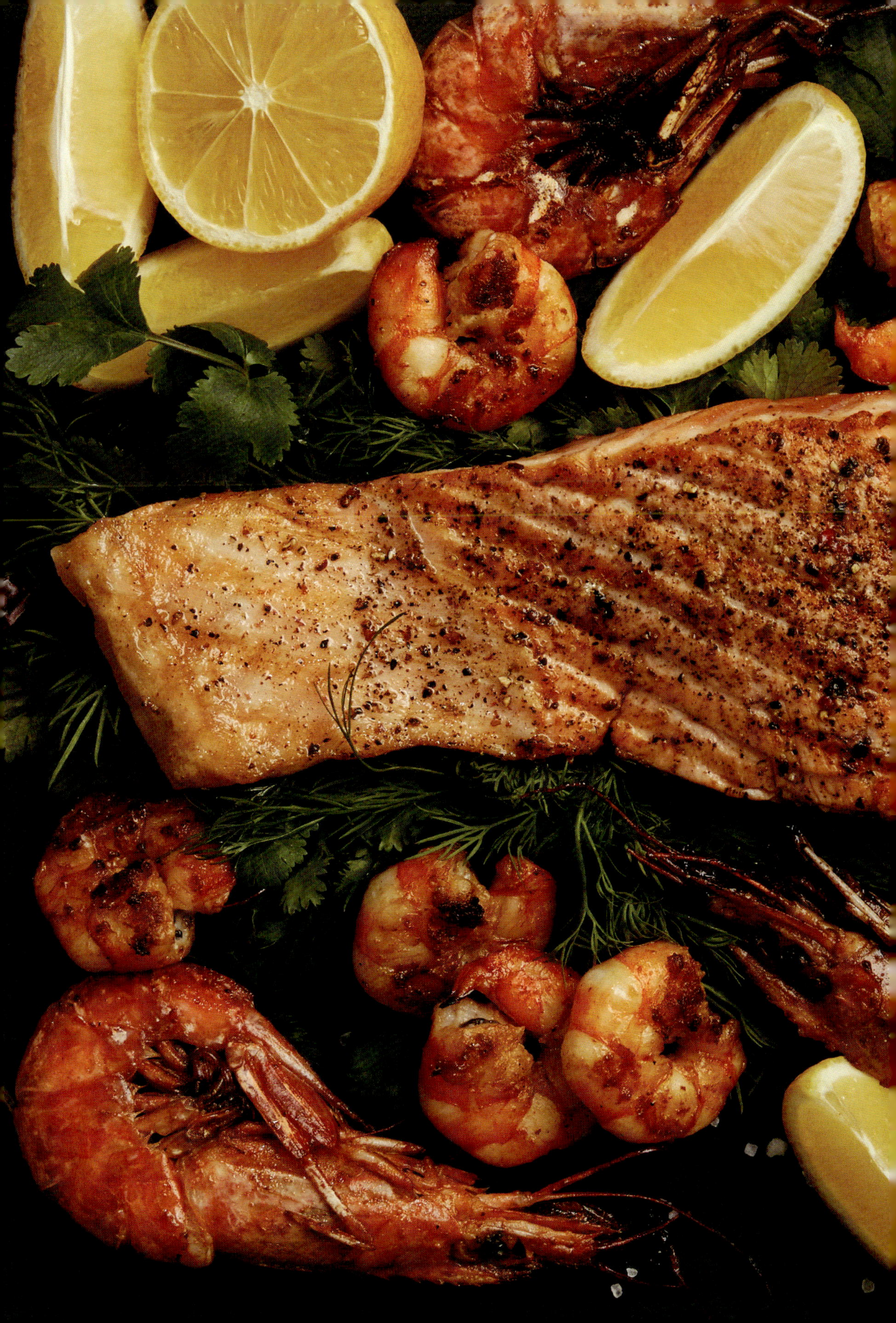

Easy fried rice

SERVES
2

Ingredients

2 cups cooked brown or white basmati rice

2 cups frozen peas, corn and carrots

3 eggs

Extra virgin olive oil

Light soy sauce or ketjap manis

Method

1. Cook rice on stove or in rice cooker
2. Cook frozen veggies or allow to thaw
3. Heat oil in pan, add veggies
4. Push to one side of pan
5. Add 3 beaten eggs and scramble in pan
6. Add cooked rice and mix together
7. Add sauce of choice and mix.

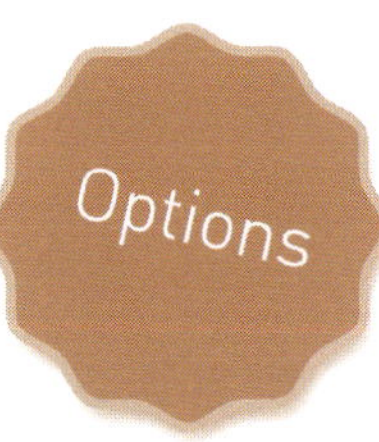

Cauliflower rice instead of brown/white rice

Slendier rice

Add any additional veggies you have

Soy sauce, oyster sauce can be used also – as these are high in sodium be sure to look for low salt varieties and use sparingly.

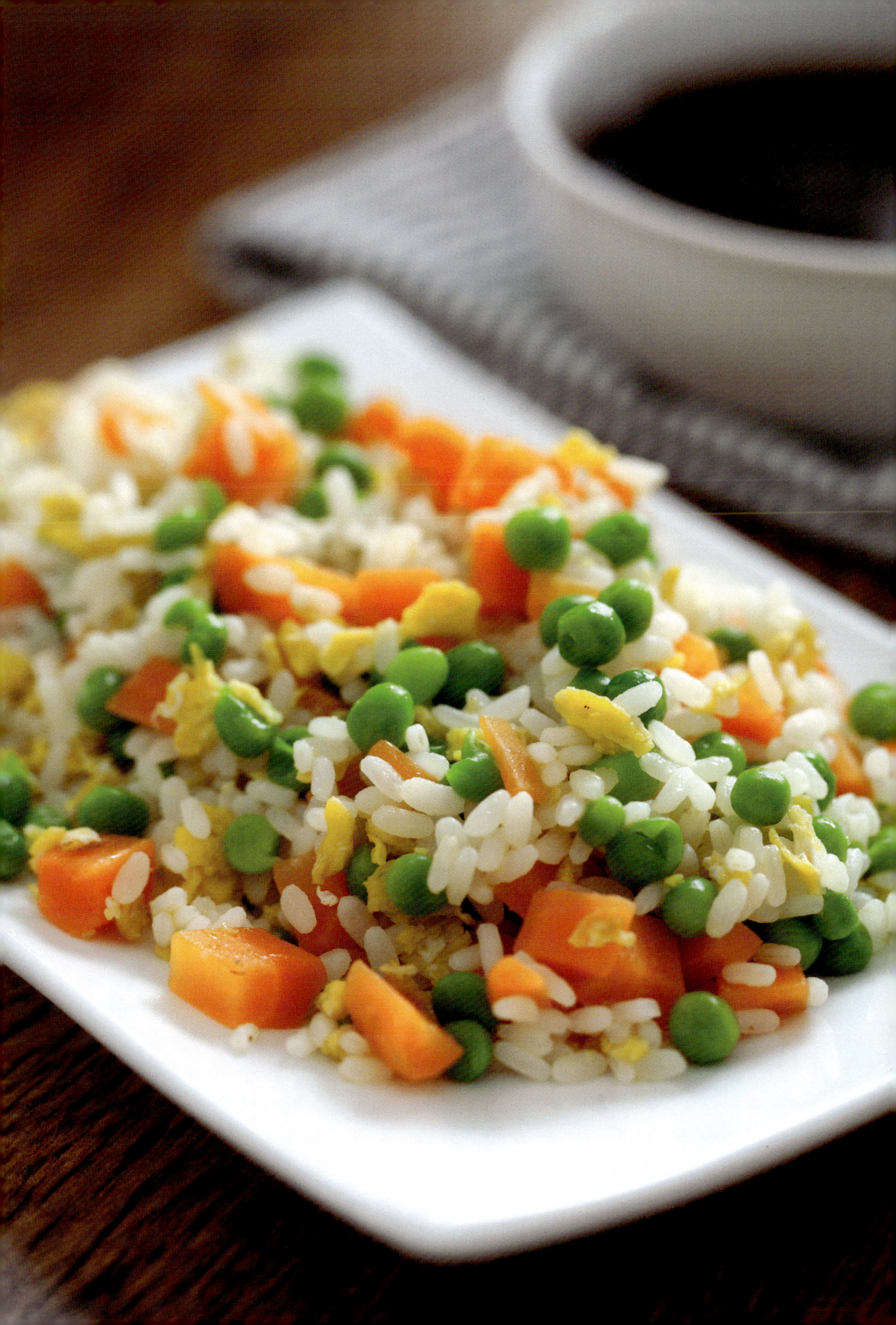

Tasting plate

We call this a mezze plate. It's simple, different and the kids love it.

Ingredients

Anything you have on hand for example:

- ham slices
- cheese cubes
- olives
- baby tomatoes
- berries
- cucumbers
- crackers

Method

Arrange on a plate and allow the family to 'pick'.

Coconut chilli vegetable curry

SERVES
2

Ingredients

3 tablespoons desiccated coconut

1 green chilli finely chopped

1cm piece of ginger finely chopped

2 garlic cloves finely chopped

2 tablespoons coconut oil

100g cauliflower chopped

100g potatoes chopped

100g peas, fresh or frozen

1 onion chopped

½ teaspoon turmeric

½ teaspoon ground coriander

100ml coconut milk

Salt and pepper

3 tablespoons fresh coriander chopped

Pinch of garam masala

Method

1. Mix the coconut, ginger, garlic and chilli together to make a paste
2. Heat the coconut oil in a heavy-based pot and add the mixture. Sauté for 1 minute
3. Add the potato, cauliflower and peas
4. Add the turmeric, coriander and season
5. After 2 minutes, add the coconut milk. Gently simmer until vegetables are just soft. Decorate with chopped coriander and top with garam masala.

San choy bow

SERVES
2

Ingredients

6 lettuce cups

200g mince of choice

½ red capsicum

¼–½ onion

½ clove garlic

1 teaspoon grated ginger

½ teaspoon chilli paste

1 teaspoon oyster sauce/ketjap manis (optional)

olive oil/sesame oil/ extra virgin olive oil spray for cooking

plain/toasted sesame seeds for garnish

Method

1. In a frypan/wok, sauté the onion, mince and capsicum in oil and spices
2. When cooked through, spoon mixture into lettuce cups
3. Garnish with toasted sesame seeds and a squeeze of lime.

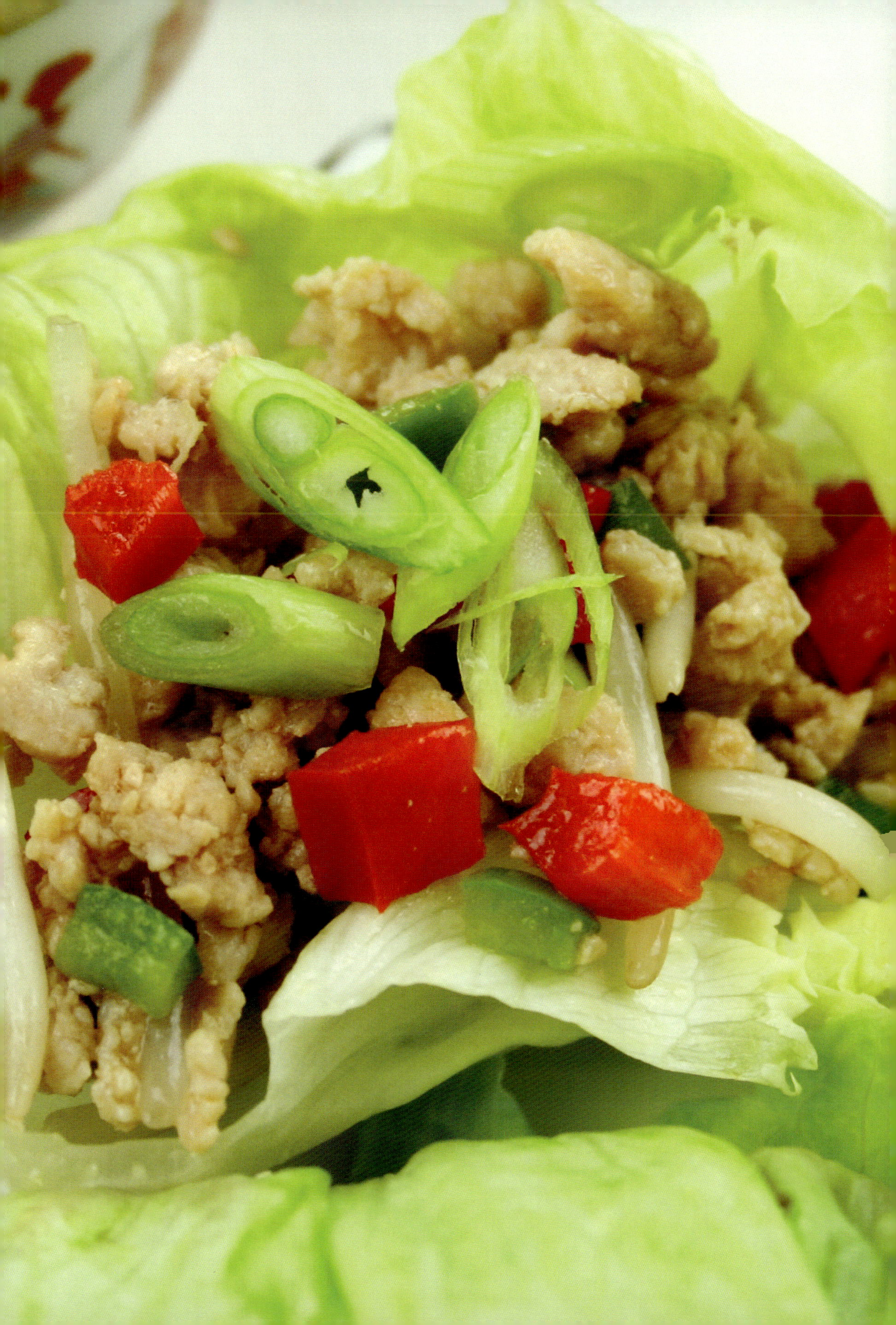

Simple stir fry Ginger and beef

SERVES
2-3

Ingredients

2 tablespoons apple cider vinegar

4 tablespoons organic soy sauce

1 tablespoon honey

3cm piece of ginger, finely chopped

2 red chillies deseeded and finely chopped

1 teaspoon ground cumin

500g beef strips

2 tablespoons coconut oil

1 Tablespoon macadamia oil

2 spring onions chopped

2 cloves garlic chopped

Method

1. Mix soy sauce, vinegar, ginger, honey, cumin, chilli in a bowl
2. Add the beef and allow to marinate for 1 hour
3. Heat oils in a wok/pan
4. Add the beef mixture, garlic and onions
5. Cook on high heat for a few minutes until beef is cooked
6. Serve with rice, salad or on some steamed green beans/other vegetable.

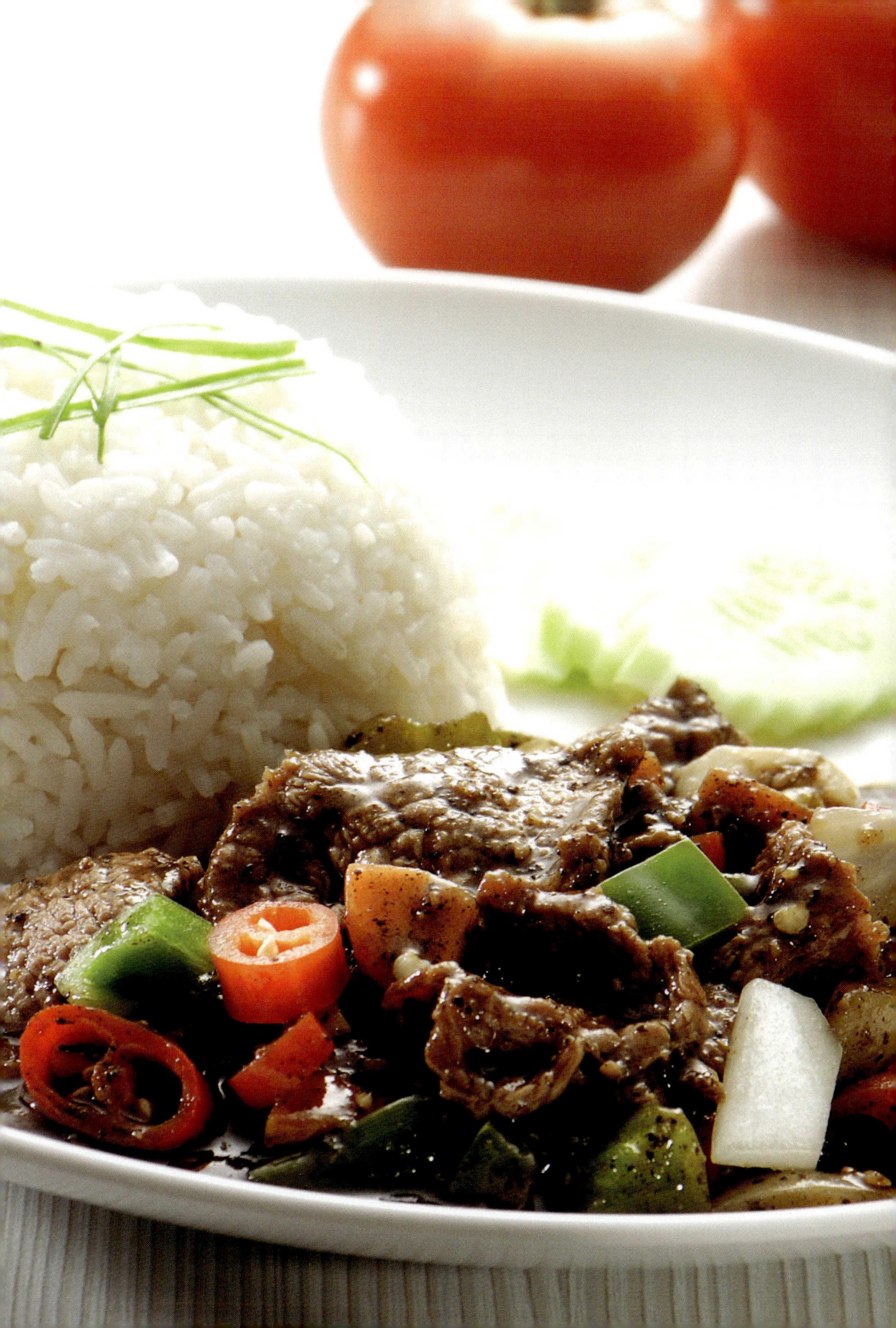

Simple stir fry
Satay chicken

SERVES
2-3

Ingredients

500g of diced chicken cut into 1cm square pieces

2 cup peanut butter/almond spread

Hot water to add to the peanut butter to form a paste

¼ cup peanuts/other nuts to garnish

1 Onion

1 Cup broccoli

1 Cup snow peas

1 Cup chopped celery

1 cup red capsicum

Method

1. Coat chicken with almond spread or peanut butter mixed with a little hot water and marinate for a couple of hours or overnight.
2. Stir fry vegetables such as red capsicum, celery, onion, snow peas, and broccoli in crushed garlic and a little coconut oil or olive oil.
3. In same pan or wok, cook the marinated chicken.
4. Add the peanuts and stir.

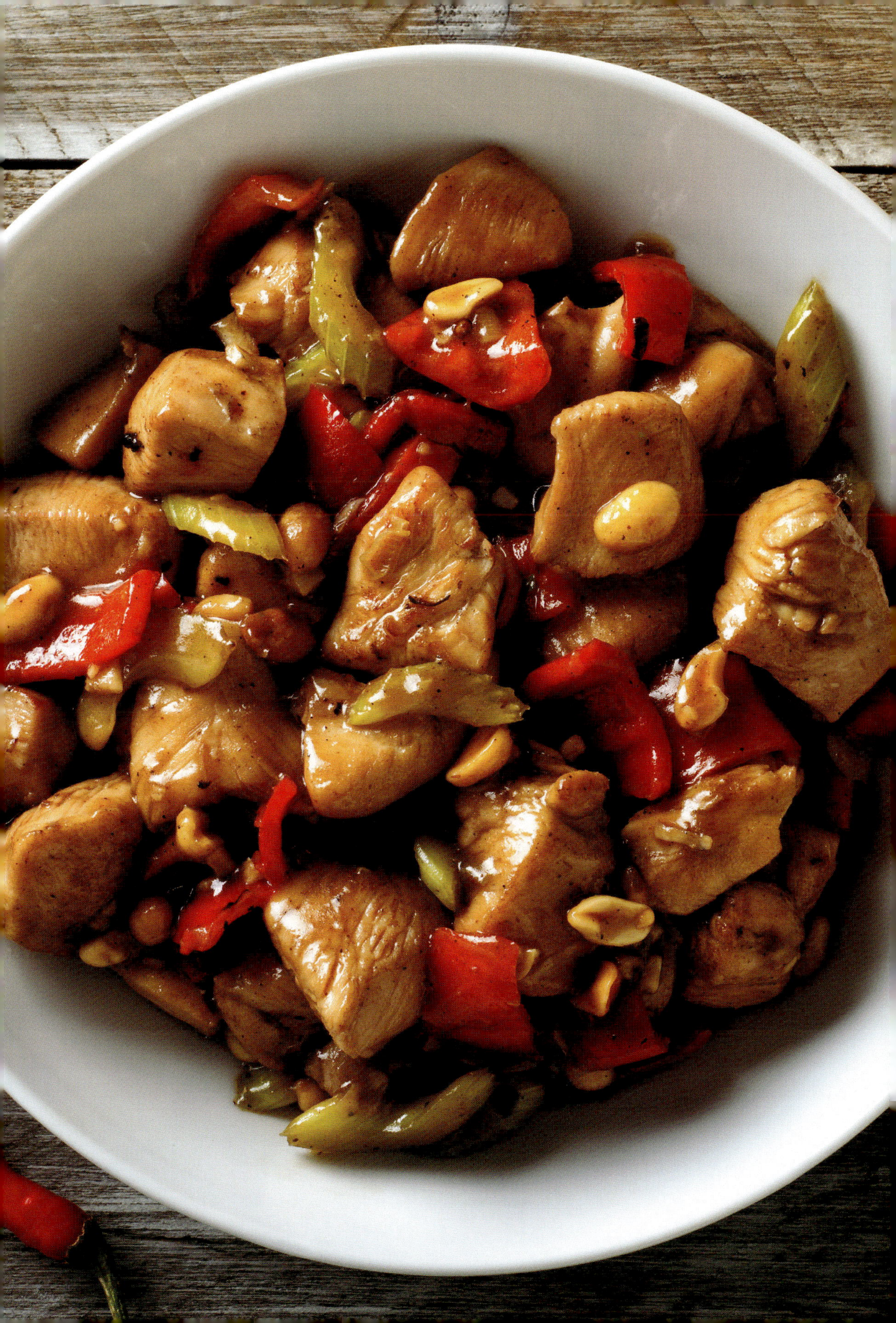

Chicken caccatorie

SERVES
4

Ingredients

6-8 skinless chicken thighs

Salt and pepper to season

2 tablespoons olive oil (more if needed)

1 medium onion diced

2 tablespoons minced garlic or 3 cloves

1 small yellow bell pepper (capsicum), diced

1 small red bell pepper (capsicum), diced medium

1 large carrot peeled and sliced

200g mushrooms sliced

½ cup pitted black olives

2 tablespoons each freshly chopped parsley and basil plus more to garnish

1 teaspoon dried oregano

150ml red wine

2 tins crushed tomatoes (820g)

4 tablespoons tomato paste

Method

1. Season chicken with salt and pepper
2. Heat oil in a heavy, cast-iron skillet, fry the onion until transparent (about 3-4 minutes) then add the garlic and sauté until fragrant (about 30 seconds)
3. Add the peppers, carrot, mushrooms and herbs, sauté for 5 minutes until vegetables are beginning to soften
4. Add the chicken and sear on both sides until golden (occasionally mix the vegetables around the chicken in the pan so they don't stick)
5. Pour in the wine; allow to simmer and reduce down (about 5-6 minutes)
6. Add the crushed tomatoes, tomato paste
7. Season with salt and pepper to taste, continue to cook on stove top OR in the oven following the instructions below
8. Mix all of the ingredients together; cover with lid, reduce heat to low and allow to simmer (while stirring occasionally) for 30-40 minutes or until the meat is cooked. Add the olives, allow to simmer for a further 10 minutes. Garnish with parsley and serve immediately.

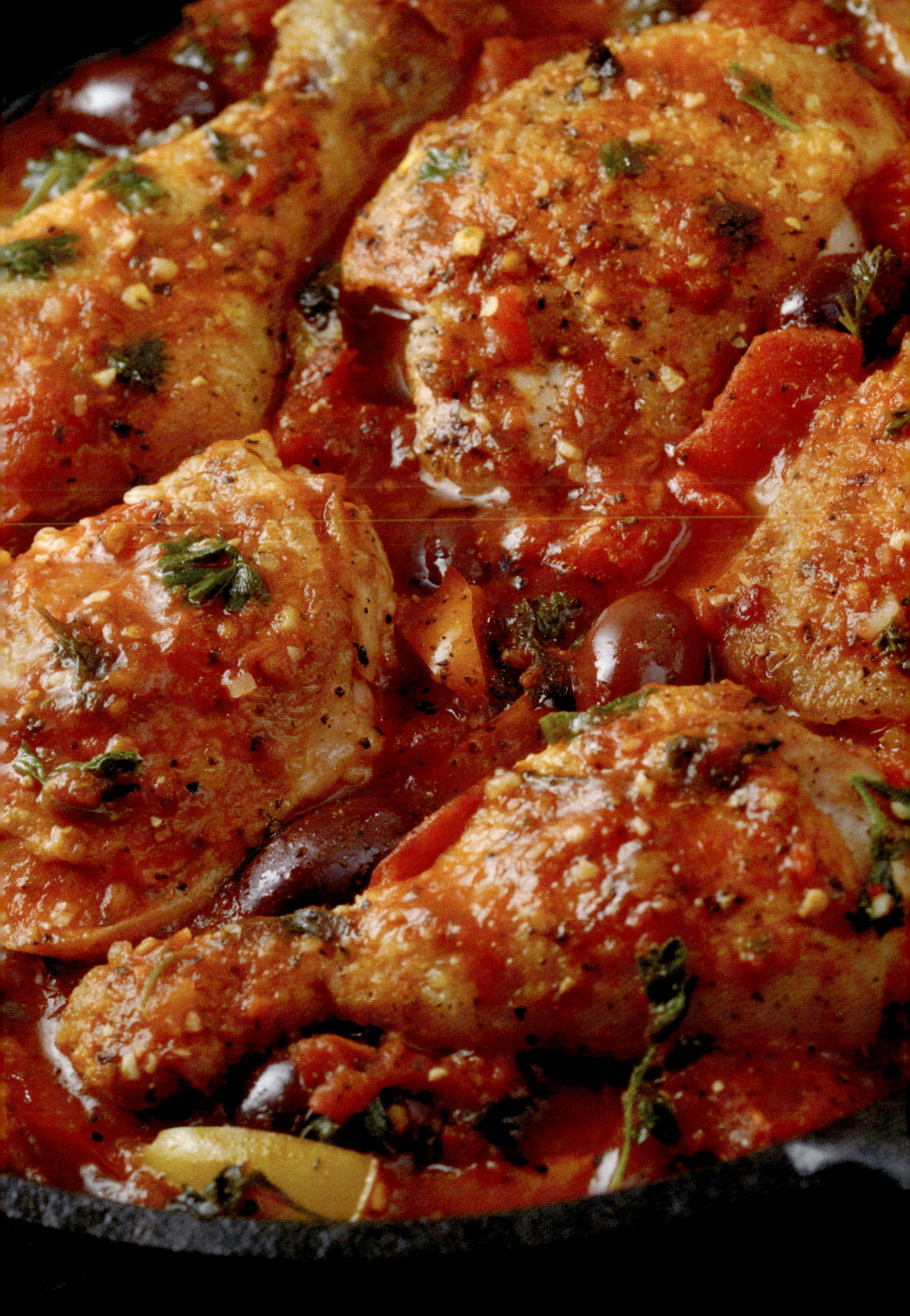

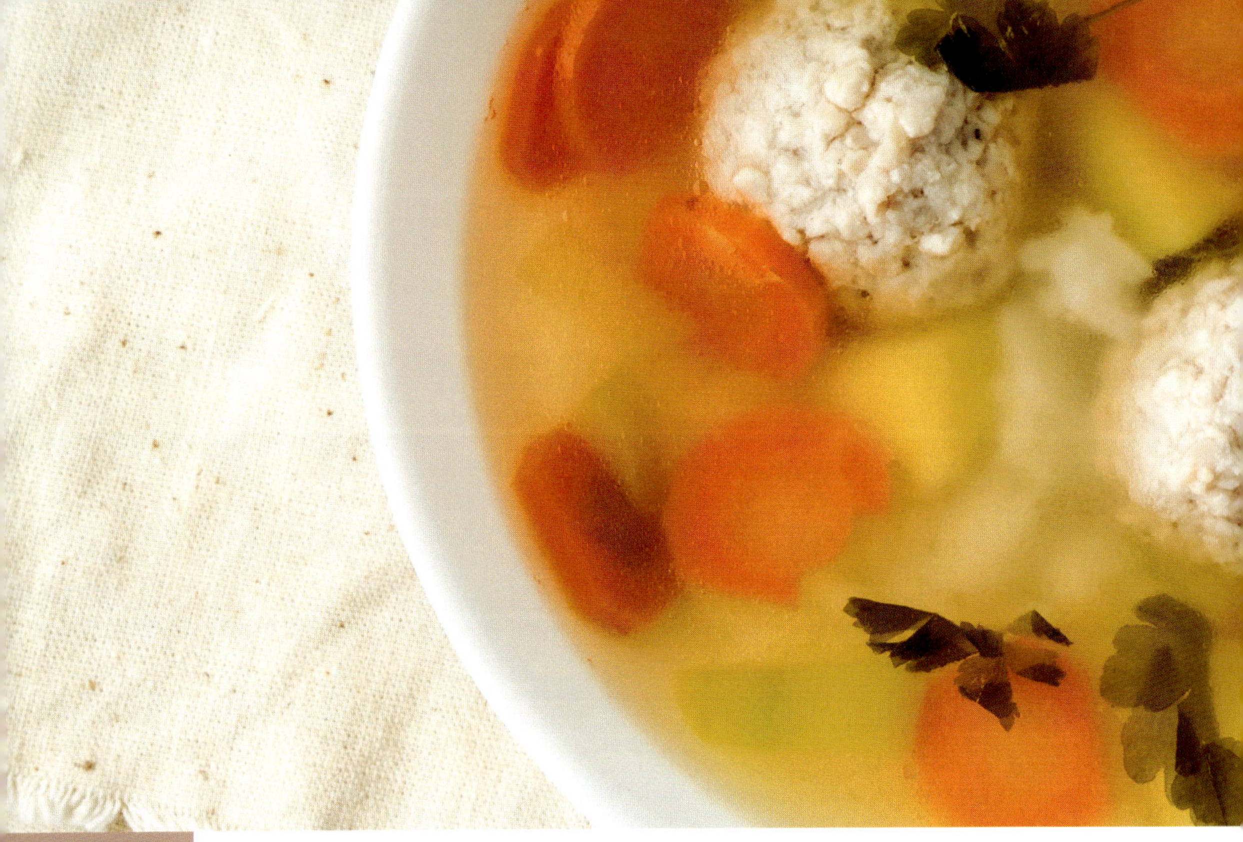

Chicken meat ball soup

SERVES
2-3

LUNCH / DINNER

I double this recipe (see note step 2) and freeze the left-over meat balls for another easy meal.

Ingredients

500g chicken mince

1 egg

¾ cup breadcrumbs (gluten free if you wish)

¾ cup grated parmesan cheese

Optional: chopped parsley if the kids don't mind the green

1-2 cloves garlic chopped

2 carrots diced

4 potatoes diced (or use sweet potato)

2 x 500ml good quality chicken stock

2litres water

3 celery sticks diced

Salt and pepper

Olive oil

Optional: crusty bread or ½ cup cooked rice

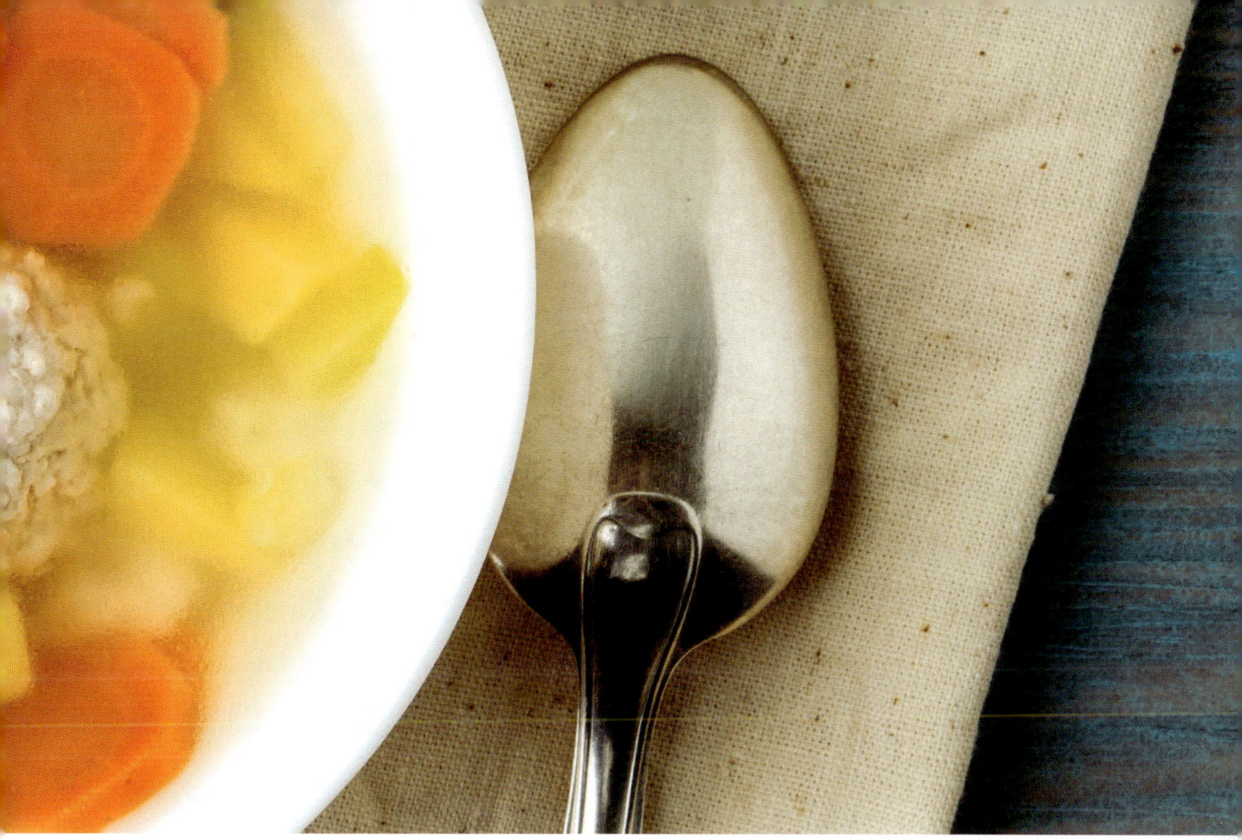

Method: Meatballs

1. Combine mince, grated parmesan, breadcrumbs and egg (and parsley if using)
2. If you're making a double quantity, just use 1 cup grated parmesan, 2 eggs and 1 cup breadcrumbs
3. Mix and roll into balls
4. Place in a separate saucepan of boiling water for just 10 mins
5. Drain and set aside to add to soup.

Method: Soup

1. Add some oil to pan/large pot then the garlic
2. Add hard veggies such as potatoes and carrots and stir fry
3. Add stock and water, you need a big pot. The liquid should be only about ¾ to the top because when you add the meatballs it will rise
4. Add celery and meatballs and bring to the boil
5. Reduce heat and simmer for about an hour on low heat.

Serve with crusty bread or cooked rice.

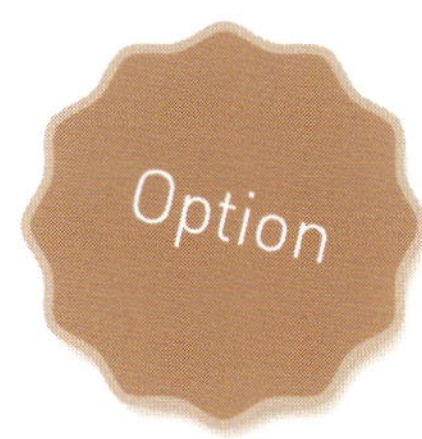

Pumpkin and cauliflower soup

SERVES
4-5

Ingredients

- 1 onion chopped
- 2 cloves of garlic
- 20g butter
- 500g pumpkin peeled and chopped
- 500g cauliflower cut into small florets
- 750ml of stock (or water plus stock cubes/homemade paste)

Method

1. Melt butter in heavy-bottom large pot, add onion and garlic and sauté until brown
2. Add pumpkin, cauliflower and water/stock
3. Bring to boil
4. Lower to simmer for 30-60 minutes until all vegetables soft
5. Blend in processor/blender until smooth consistency.

Serve with bread and or protein side of choice.

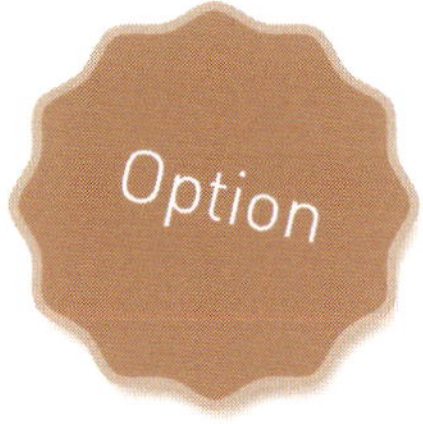

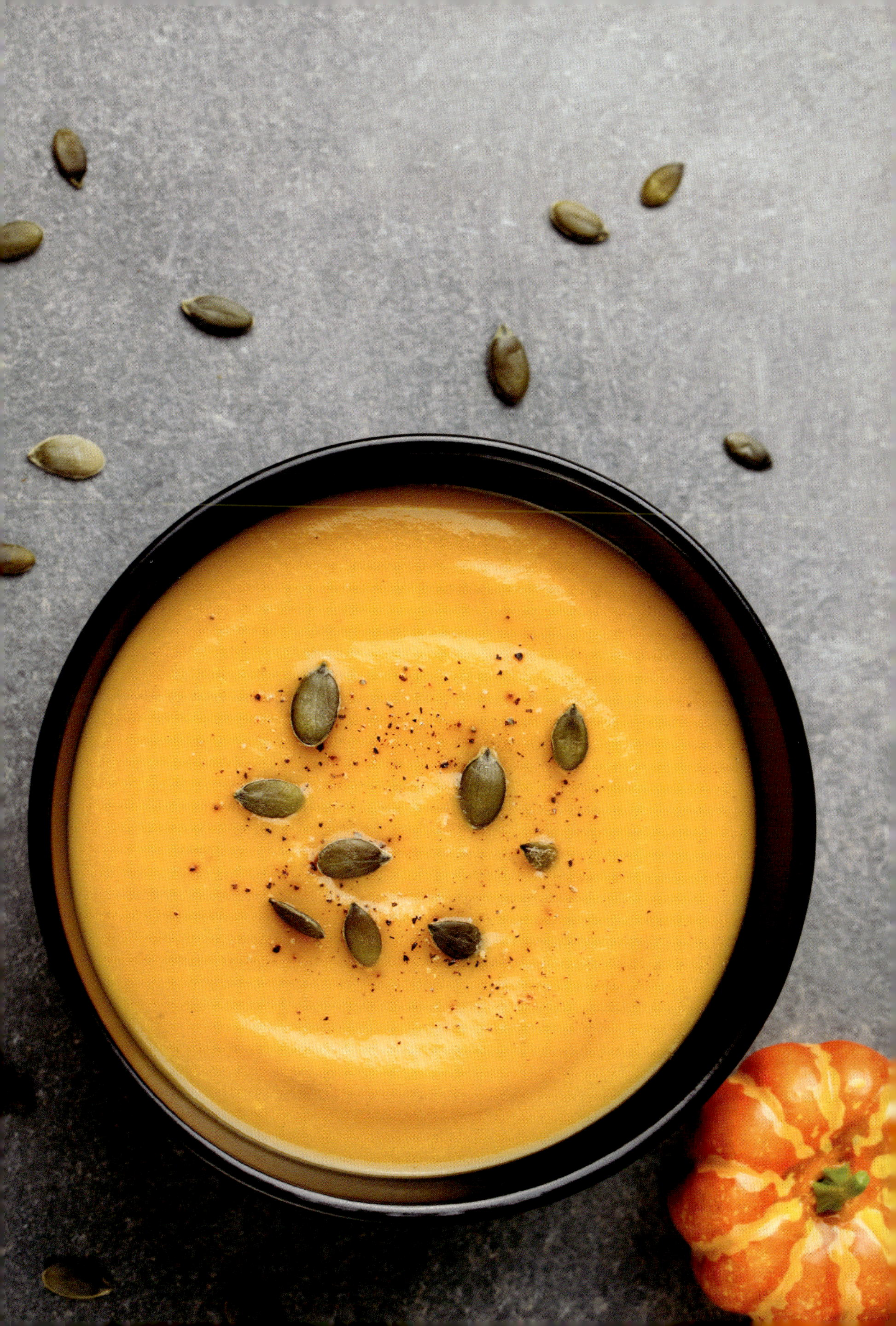

Chocolate mousse

SERVES
2

Ingredients

2 ripe avocados
½ cup cacao
½ tablespoon vanilla extract
3 tablespoons raw honey
2 tablespoons coconut oil
½ cup water

Method

1. Mash avocado with fork
2. Blend or stir to combine avocado with all other ingredients
3. Add water as needed until desired consistency is reached.
4. Refrigerate to set.

Add ½ cup desiccated coconut to taste.

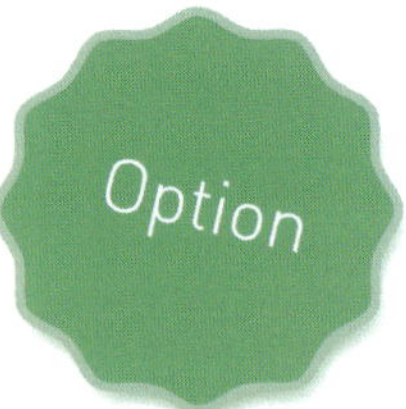

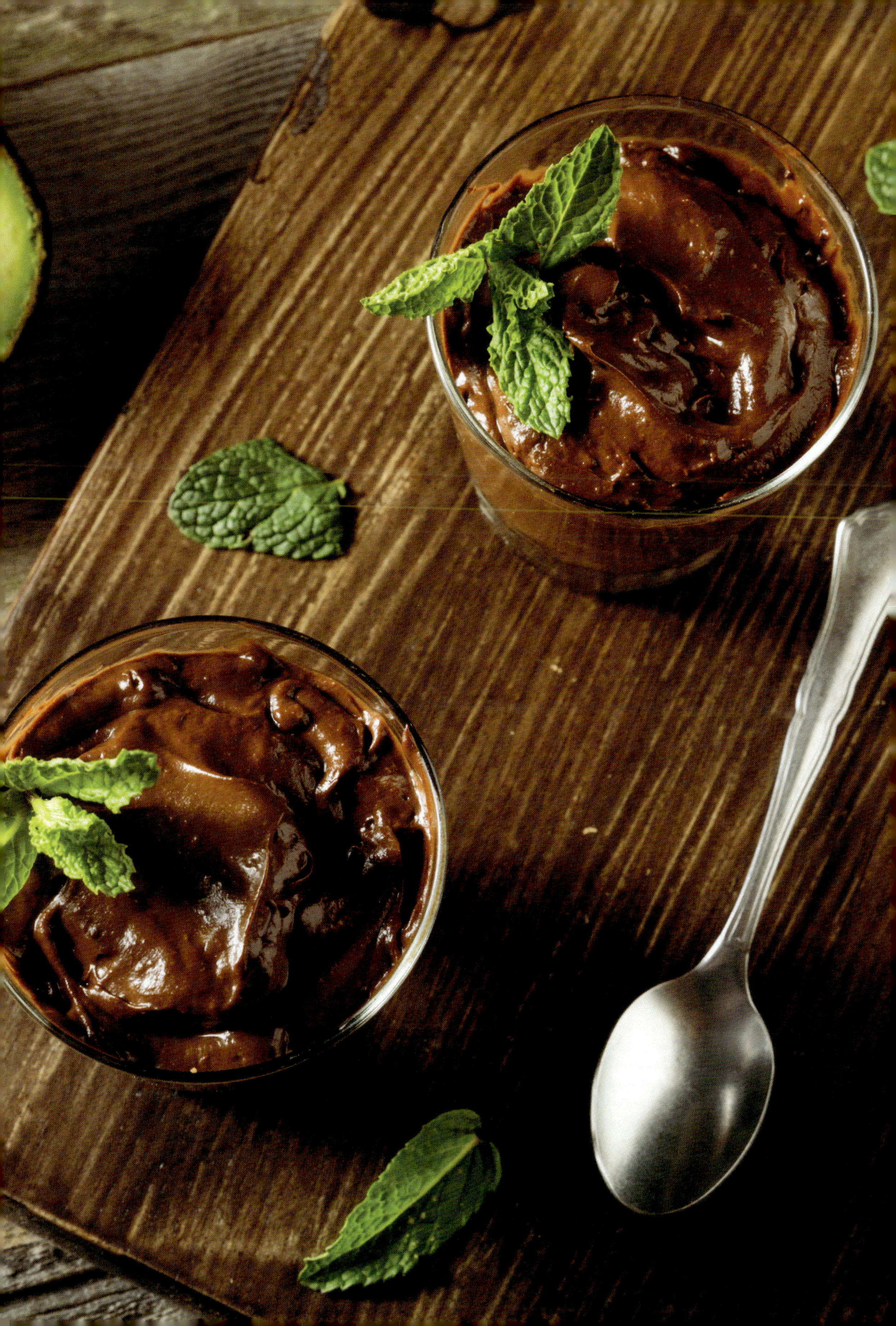

Apple crumble

SERVES
4-6

This gluten free crumble is a great accompaniment to yoghurt or ice cream.

Or it can be a sweeter indulgence for breakfast as a granola with some fresh fruit and/or almond milk.

Ingredients

Apple

Boil or bake apple whole/pieces until soft (No sugar or sweetener needed), or cut apple up and bake as a pie.

Crumble

- ½ cup almond meal
- 1½ teaspoons cinnamon
- 1 cup shredded coconut
- ⅔ cup walnuts chopped
- 1 egg white
- 50g organic melted butter
- 1-2 tablespoons melted raw honey (add after cooking)

Method

1. Mix dry ingredients together
2. Add and stir through egg white (to bind) and butter
3. Press out and flatten on baking paper
4. Bake 20-30 minutes until golden
5. Once cooked, melt honey for a few seconds in microwave; drizzle honey over the crumble (do this after cooking so the sweetness isn't lost)
6. Loosen and separate crumble. Store in container in the fridge once cooled.
7. Serve over ½ a baked apple with some plain yoghurt or occasionally a single scoop of vanilla ice cream.

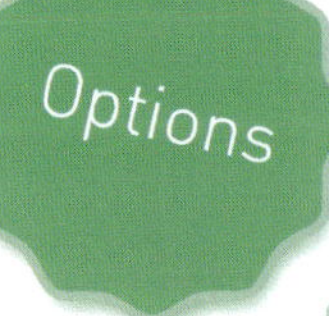

Replace apple with other baked/stewed fruit of choice

Can use crumble as toasted muesli alternative with fruit and yoghurt for breakfast.

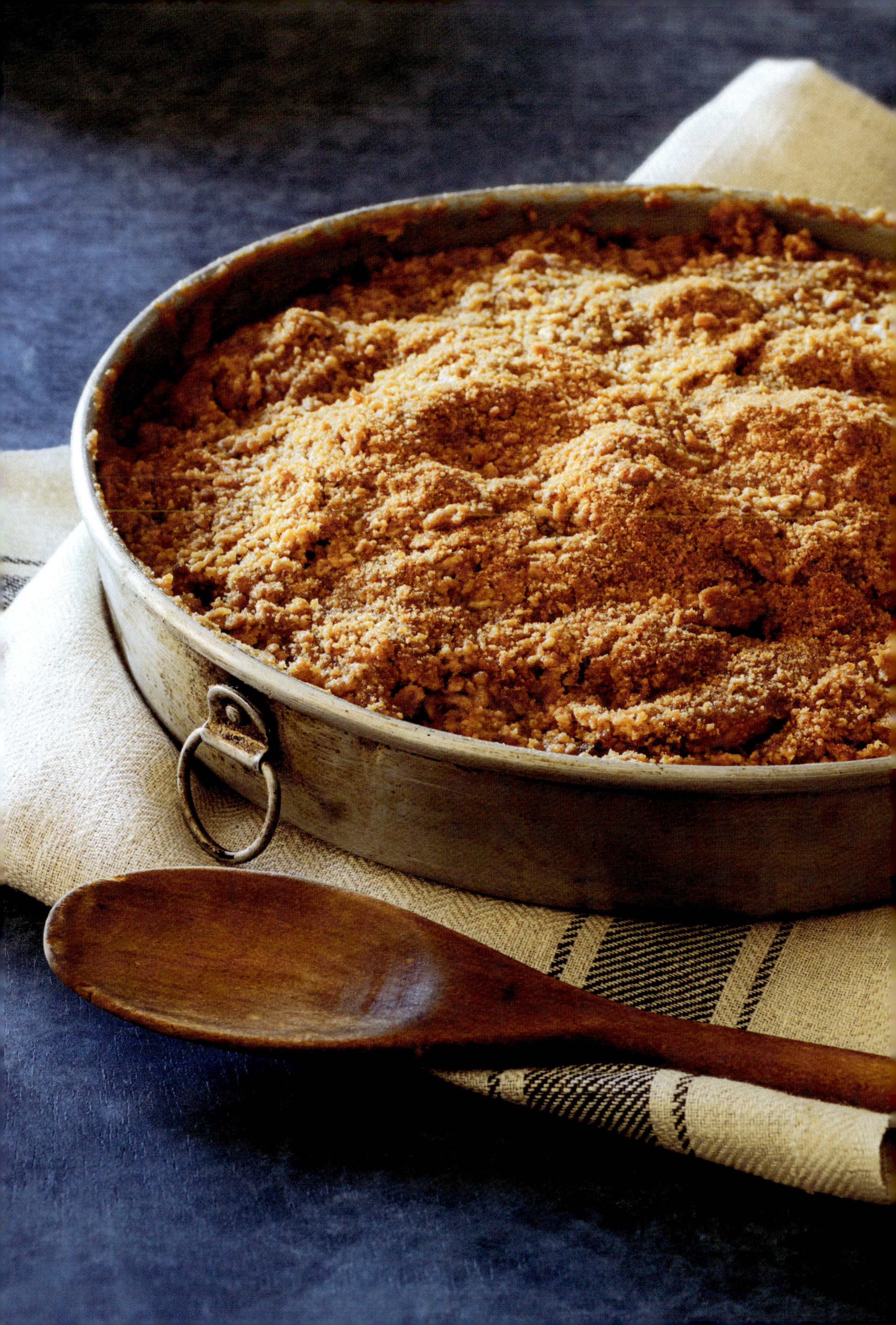

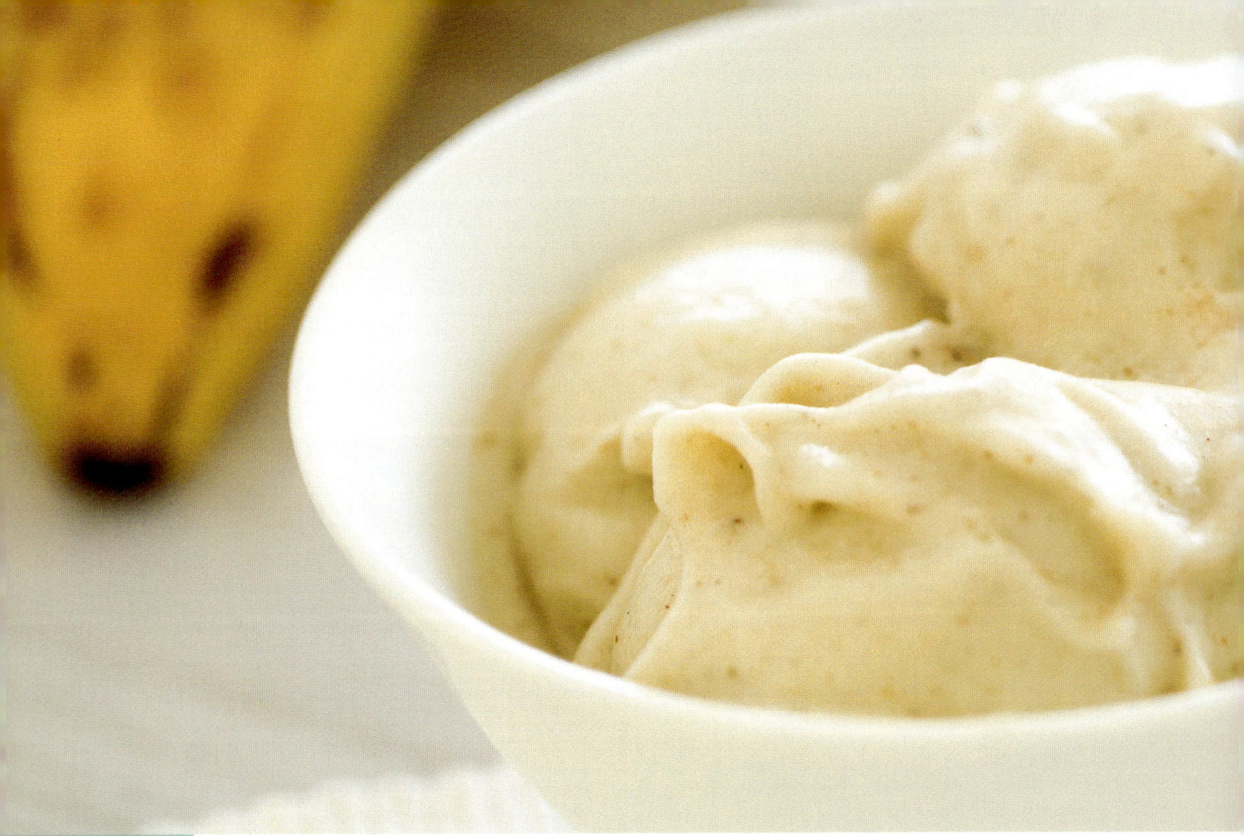

Homemade ice cream

SERVES
3

This ice cream topped with crunchy muesli, granola or crumble is delicious!

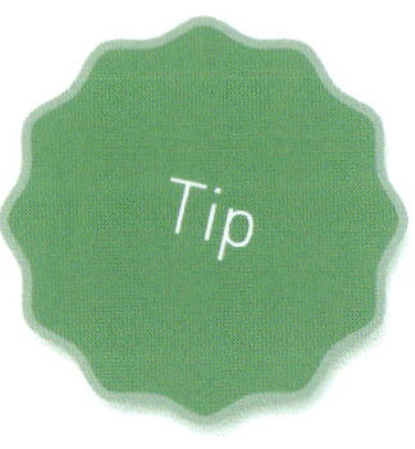

→ See recipes on pages 66, 68, and 150

DESSERT

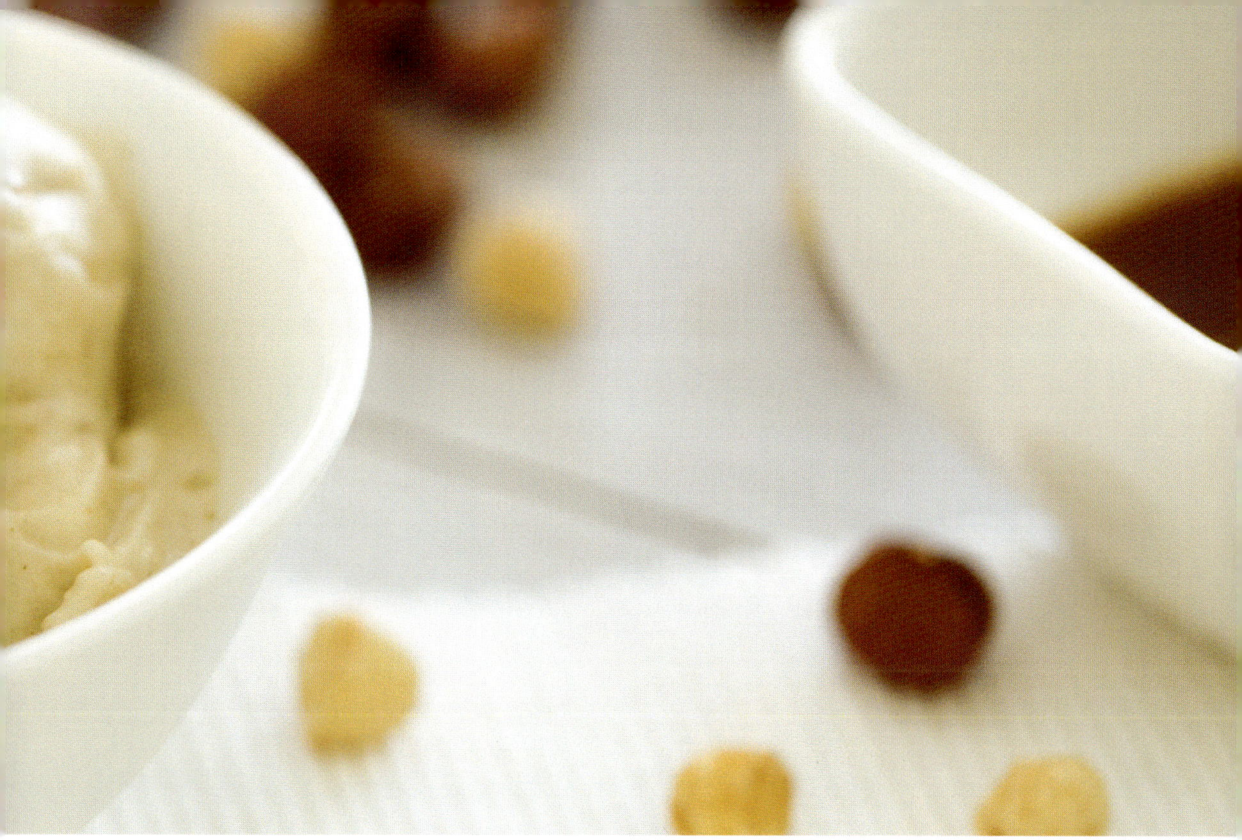

Ingredients

250g frozen banana

½ cup almond milk

To add flavour such as almonds, chocolate chips, milo, cacao or peanut butter, please add these ingedients at step 1.

Method

1. Place frozen banana and almond milk in blender
2. Blitz until a smooth consistency
3. Serve immediately or freeze for an hour before serving to allow it to harden a little

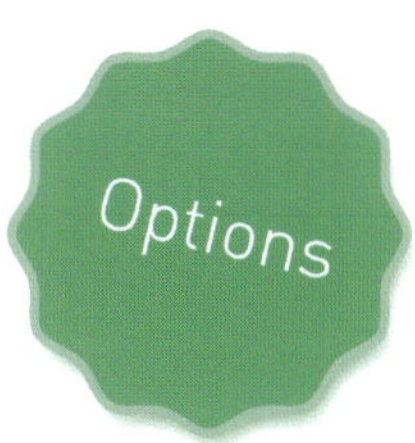

Add ½ cup chopped roasted almonds or pecans plus 1 tablespoon almond butter

Add some chopped dark chocolate (any flavour) or choc chips

Add some raw cacao powder (or Milo for the kids).

Ice pops
Watermelon

Ingredients

Watermelon

Method

1. Place pieces of watermelon in blender with a little water until liquid consistency
2. Pour into popsicle moulds and freeze.

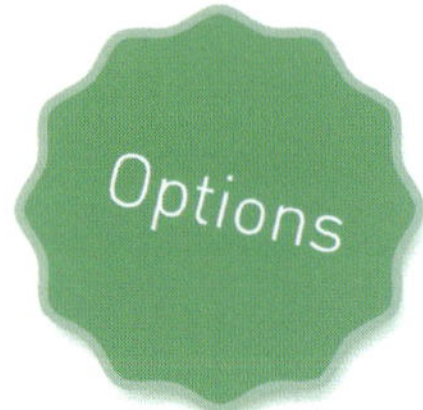

You can do this with any fruit

Add water if needed to get the right consistency.

DESSERT

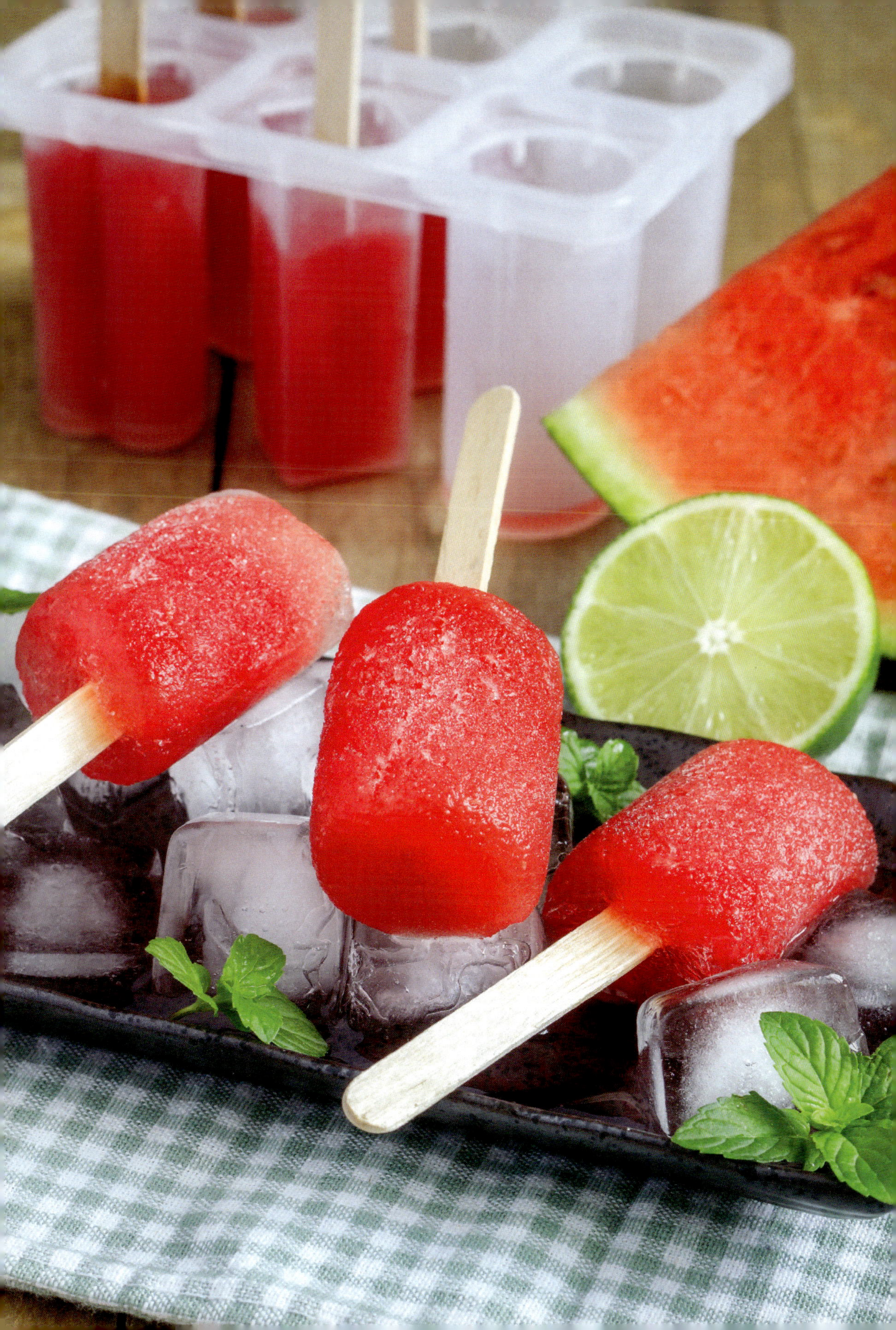

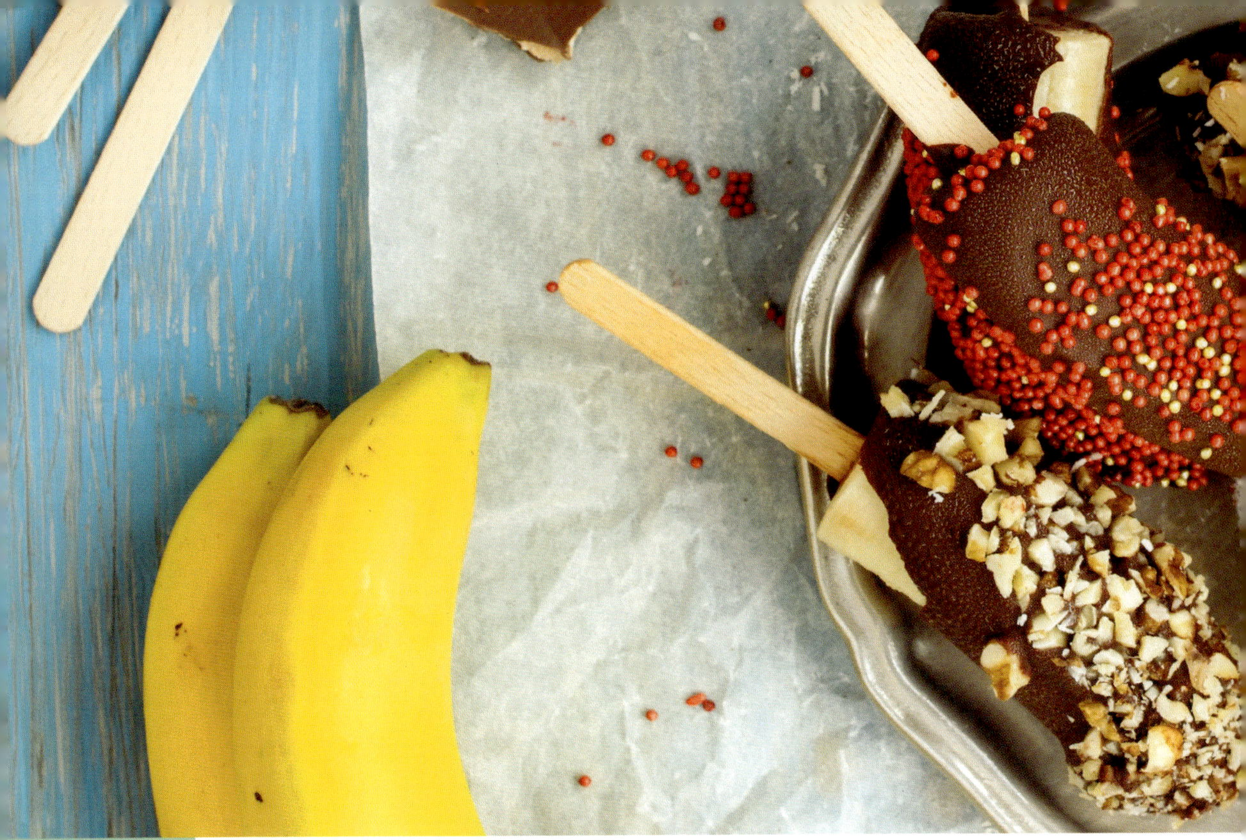

Ice pops Banana

SERVES 3

Kids love making these!

Surprisingly, they taste exactly like a Paddle Pop

Kids can make these themselves and use their fave topping such as chopped chocolate, Milo or some sprinkles

You can also do these as ice cream bites. Cut bananas into bite sizes and follow instructions above.

For peanut butter and banana bites cut two wedges of banana and spread peanut butter/ almond spread through the middle, then dip in chocolate, place on baking paper and freeze for an hour.

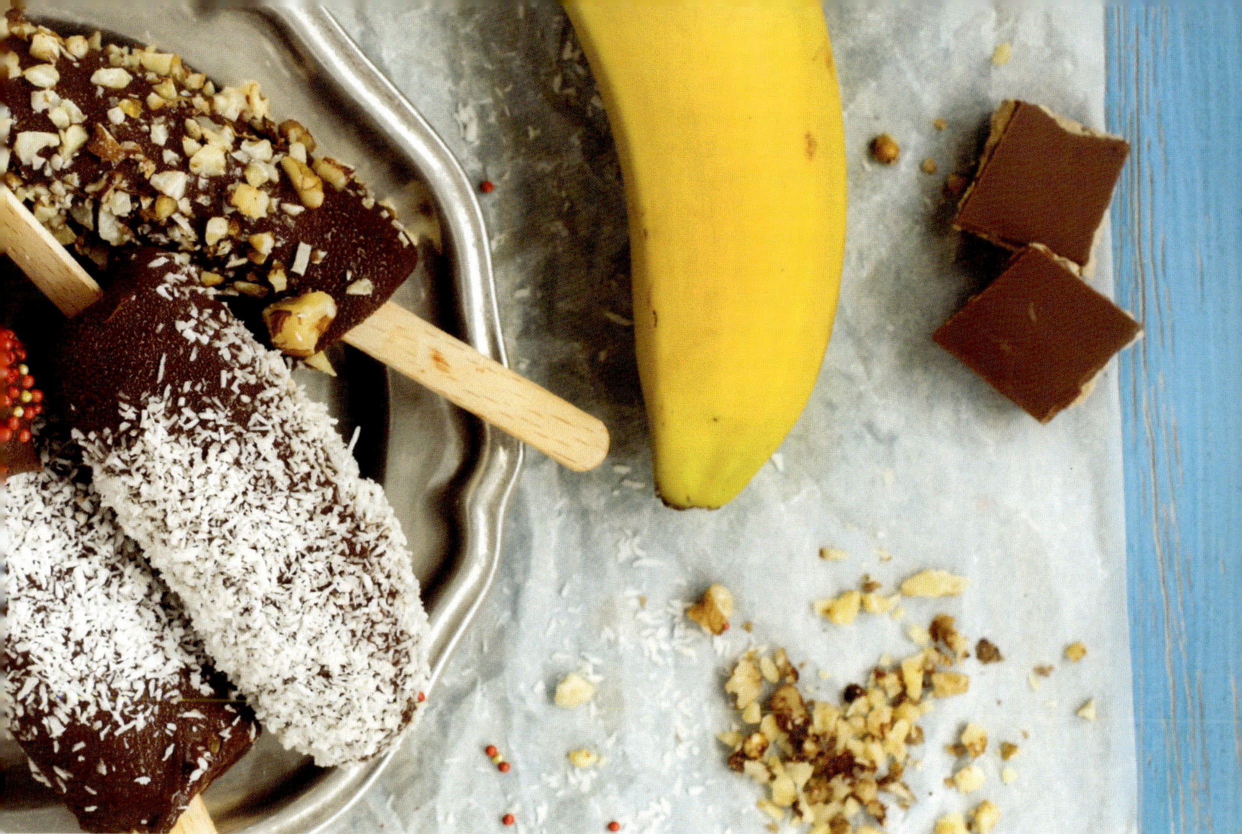

Ingredients

Small bananas

Melted dark or milk chocolate

Nuts, coconut, or sprinkles for topping

Method

1. Melt chocolate
2. Place Paddle Pop stick in banana
3. Gently dip into chocolate
4. Coat in topping of choice
5. Place on baking paper and freeze for an hour.

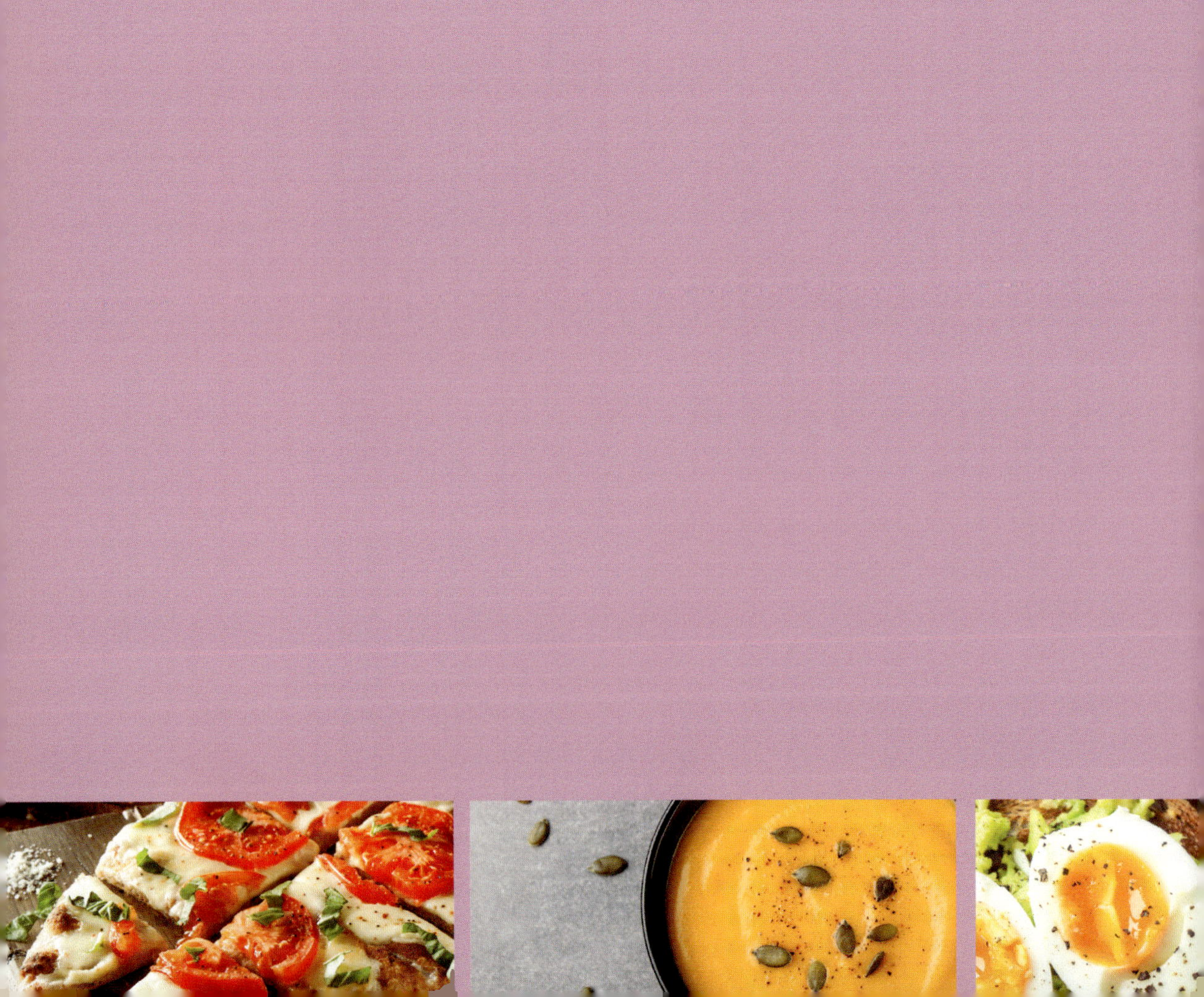

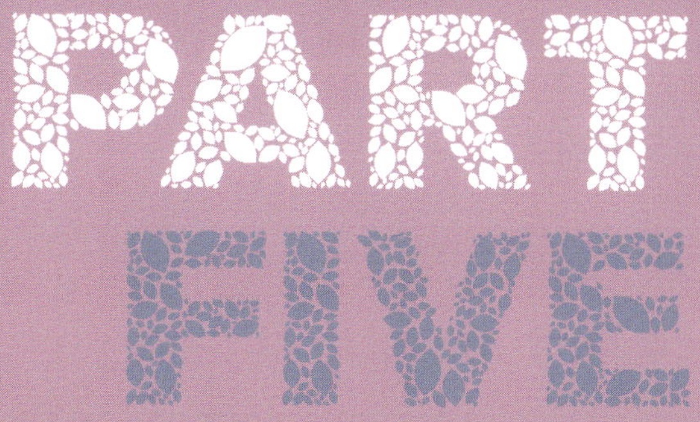

Family menu plan

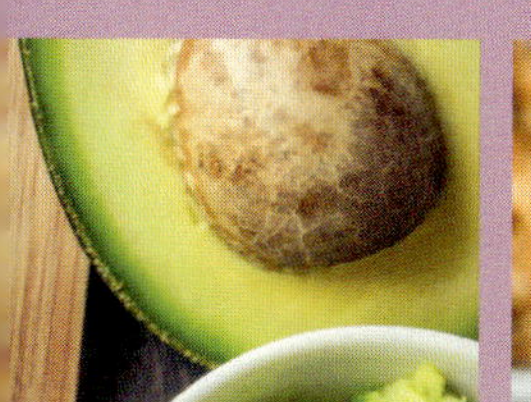
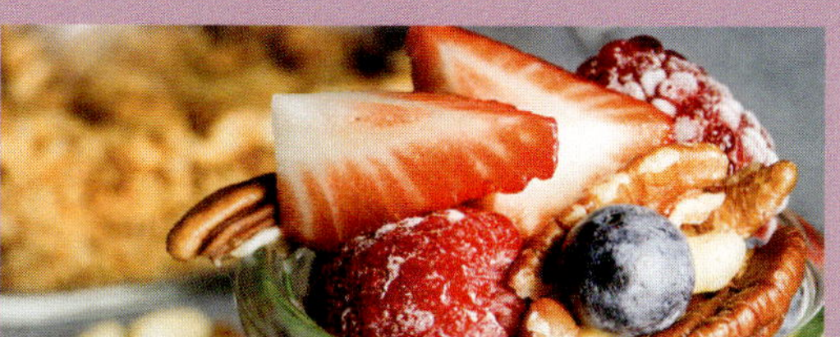
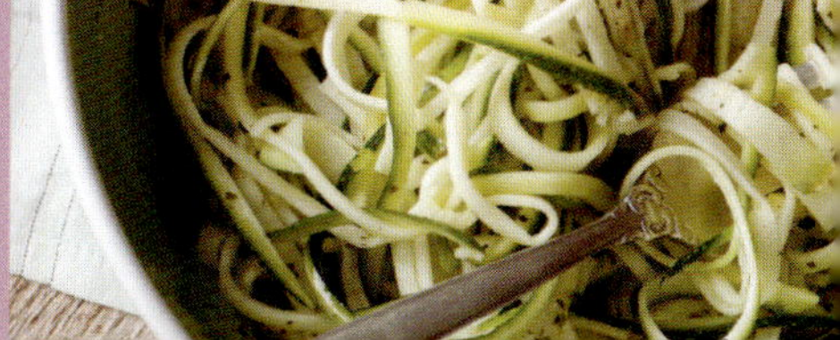

	MONDAY	TUESDAY	WEDNESDAY
Breakfast	Omelette	Homemade muesli	Smashed avocado with egg
Morning tea	Raw veggies sticks with avocado dip	Egg muffin	Seeded crackers with hommus
Lunch	Wrap	Sweet potato and walnut salad	Rice paper rolls
Afternoon tea	Muffin	Raw veggies sticks/celery boats with nut butter	Nuts and seeds
Dinner	Sweet potato and fetta pie	San choy bow with mince	Crumbed baked chicken
After dinner	Herbal tea	Herbal tea	Herbal tea
Notes			

	THURSDAY	FRIDAY	SATURDAY	SUNDAY
	Smoothie	Peanut butter on toast	Eggs and sides	Buckwheat pancakes
	Muffin	Egg muffin	Muesli bar slice	Handful raw nuts and seeds
	Rice salad	Fritters and salad	Wrap	Two egg muffins
	Muesli slice	Bliss ball	Raw veggies sticks/celery boats with nut butter	Banana bread
	Tuna balls and salad	Stir fry	Burger and chips	Pumpkin and cauliflower soup
	Herbal tea	Herbal tea	Herbal tea	Herbal tea

Pantry

The staples

Herbs and spices

- Basil
- Pepper
- Chilli flakes
- Cinnamon
- Dukkah
- Cumin
- Coriander
- Garlic ginger
- Nutmeg
- Parsley
- Oregano
- Turmeric
- Pink Himalayan salt
- Iodized salt

TIPS

- Clear out the pantry of all processed and refined sugar products.
- Shop weekly so you never have too much temptation on hand.
- Use a farmers market if you can to purchase produce. It will be fresh, cheaper and last longer.
- Find a health food store that can supply you with specialty items.
- Make your own foods as much as possible.
- A weekend cook up of frittata, boiled eggs, bliss balls etc will ensure you have convenient food on hand.
- Grow your herbs or other produce. Fresh is best!

Nuts and seeds

- Sesame
- Pepita
- Sunflower
- All raw nuts
- Almond meal

Cooking and other

- Shredded/desiccated/flaked coconut
- Bicarb of soda
- Dates
- Goji berries
- Cacao
- Vanilla
- Peppermint essence/oil
- Extra virgin olive oil
- Coconut oil
- Butter
- Apple cider vinegar
- Balsamic vinegar
- Seeded mustard
- Honey
- Mayonnaise (the real stuff)
- Low sodium soy/ketchup manis

Tinned stuff

- Tuna/salmon
- Diced tomatoes
- Tomato paste
- Corn
- Four-bean mix
- Chickpeas
- Lentils

Products

- Low-carb pizza base/ muffins/bread mix by PBCo. (The Protein Bread Company: www.lovepbco.com)
- Slendier noodles/rice

Exercise

At home body weight and free weight exercises for the older teens and adults.

Going for a walk is the simplest exercise to do. You can take the dog, walk as a family, or walk at your own pace. There is no need for expensive gym memberships. With a few pieces of equipment, a home workout is easy!

Combining body weight, free weights and cardio into your exercise regime is great for variety and long-term results.

Kids of all ages should be walking, riding their bike, having active play in the backyard, park or pool. Body weight exercises and some healthy competition with your siblings will make movement fun. For example, who can skip the longest or do the most push-ups.

Kids can also join structured exercise groups such as boot camp where exercise is fun and interactive. Exercises are simple, progressive and a great way to make friends.

NOTE

All these exercises can be modified to suite the age of your children.

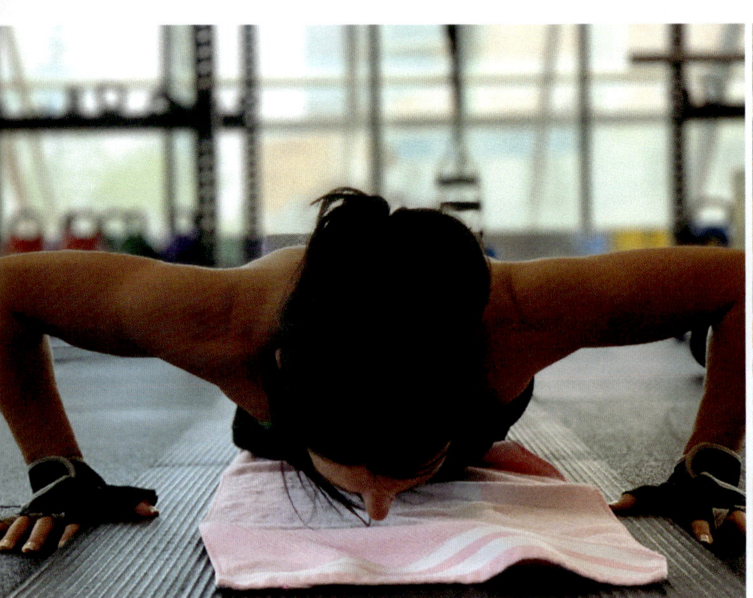

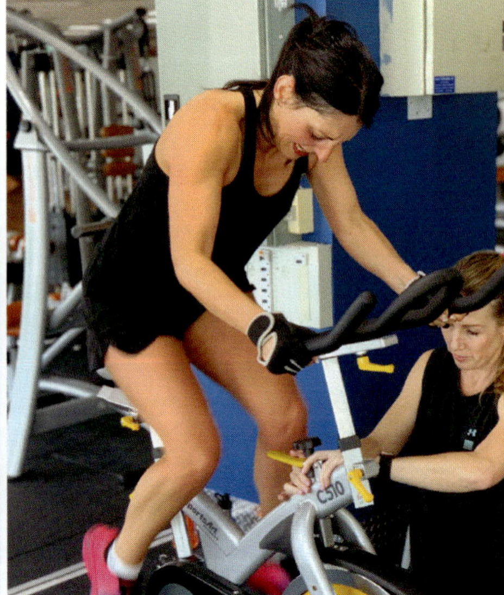

Weekly exercise plan	
MONDAY	Walk one hour at moderate pace
TUESDAY	• Body weight exercises at home • Walking up stairs (every second stair) x 10 • Dips off a chair x 20 • Sit-ups x 12 • Push-ups x 10 • Walking lunges x 10 Repeat 3-4 rounds or about 30 minutes total.
WEDNESDAY	Walk at moderate to brisk pace
THURSDAY	• Dumbbell shoulder press • Squats with kettle bell • Kettle bell up right row • Dumbbell rows • Lateral raises • Medicine ball good mornings Aim for 8-12 repetitions for each exercise. Repeat 3-4 rounds or about 30-40 minutes total.
FRIDAY	Walking at a brisk pace
SATURDAY	• Circuit training with Tuesday or Thursday exercises • Skip x 100 • Kettle bell squat x 12 • Push-ups x 12 • Walking lunges with dumbbell, medicine ball or kettle bell x 10 • Dips x 20 • Mountain climbers x 20 • Medicine ball over the shoulder x 10 Repeat for 30-40 minutes
SUNDAY	Rest

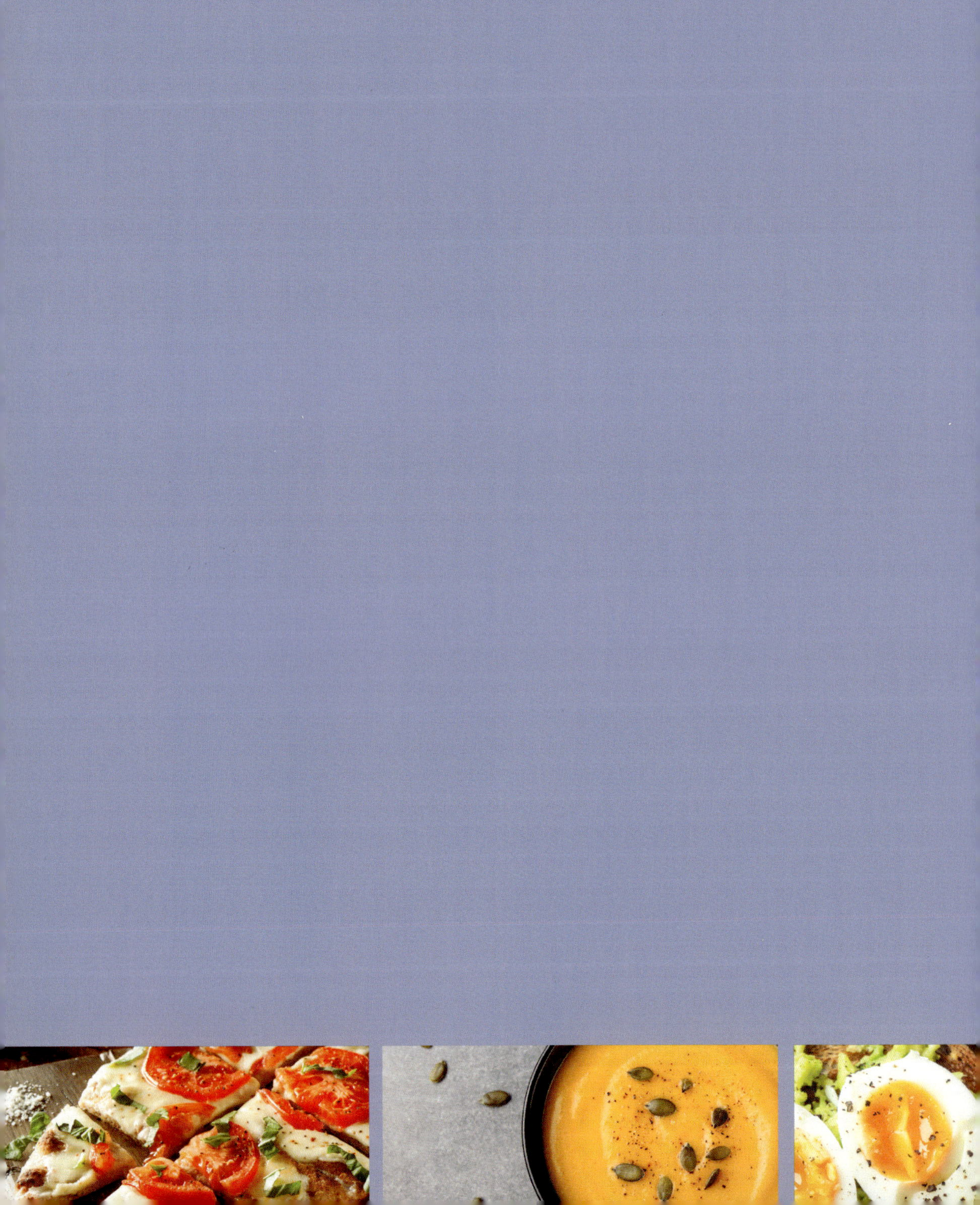

APPENDICES

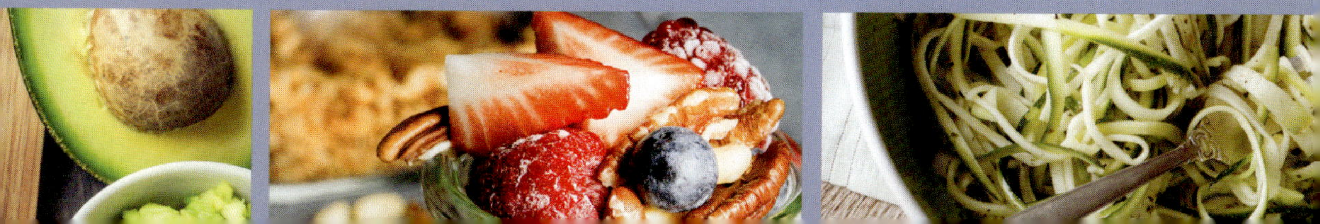

Herbs and spices

Herbs and Spices to Boost Your Metabolism

Herbs and spices have been used for centuries to enhance the flavour and nutrition of food – in addition to providing medicinal benefits. You can really enhance the flavour of food such as sauces, marinades, dressings and soups, casseroles, and stir-fry with herbs and spices. In fact, any dish can be improved with the addition of spices or herbs. I'm not just talking about hot spices; there are many spices that are not 'hot' which you can use to enrich the flavour of your food and add healthy flavonoids to your meal. Herbs usually come from the leaves of plants, while spices come from different parts of the plant; for example: berries – peppercorn; buds – cloves; seeds – cumin; bark – cinnamon; roots – ginger.

Most spices and herbs provide calcium, iron, magnesium, phosphorus, potassium, sodium, zinc, copper, manganese, and selenium in addition to Vitamin A, C, E and B complex vitamins such as thiamine, riboflavin, niacin, pantothenic acid, pyridoxine, and folate. The phytochemicals in herbs and spices have many health-giving properties. For example: they are powerful antioxidants, reduce inflammation and free radicals, and help fight bacterial infections. For example: curcumin in turmeric and capsaicin in chilli are powerful anti-inflammatory chemicals. Allin in garlic reduces blood pressure. Many herbs and spices are used in traditional remedies to help treat all sorts of disorders from nausea to infections to gout.

TIP

To get the full benefit of herbs, you should eat them fresh. The easiest and cheapest way is to grow your own herbs in the kitchen, garden or on your balcony. Seeds should be bought from organic seed growers rather than hardware chains, as these seedlings come with growth hormones and may possibly be GM strains.

When you cut fresh herbs and pop them straight into a casserole or salad, you get the full benefit of the nutrients. Compare that to a jar of dried herbs, which has been in the cupboard for a year and probably has very few nutrients left. Possibly the worst thing to have happened to herbs is the supermarket giving them a two-year sell-by date. This means that they've been sitting there losing their nutrients for a very long time.

Rosemary	is useful for stimulating the immune system, increasing circulation, and improving digestion. Rosemary also contains anti-inflammatory compounds, which have anti-fungal and antiseptic properties.
Parsley	is rich in Vitamin A, C, B1 and B6. It contains beta-carotene, iron, calcium, and magnesium. Parsley is effective for acidic urine, menstrual problems, and fluid retention.
Cinnamon	has anti-inflammatory properties and increases blood flow to vital organs. It has also been used to control blood sugar levels in diabetics.
Turmeric	is a rich orange spice that really packs a punch. It contains curcumin, a powerful phytonutrient, which has antioxidant and anti-inflammatory properties.
Garlic	protects our cells from damage caused by free radicals. It contains allin, which is a great anti-inflammatory phytonutrient.
Basil	Thai basil, or sweet basil, is common in Mediterranean cooking. It is great with tomatoes and pairs well with parmesan, oil and pine nuts as a pesto.
Nutmeg	is the dried nut of an evergreen tree. It has strong antioxidant properties and contains many phytonutrients.
Ginger	is a common ingredient in Asian cuisine. Ginger is beneficial for relieving digestive problems such as nausea, loss of appetite, motion sickness and pain. It also helps reduce inflammation and treat inflammatory conditions.
Oregano	is used to treat respiratory tract disorders, gastrointestinal disorders, menstrual cramps and urinary tract disorders. It has also been used to control acne and dandruff. It has high levels of Vitamin K, antioxidants, and has anti-inflammatory and antibacterial properties.
Chillies	contain capsaicin which promotes the release of chemicals that increase heart rate and trigger endorphins to give you a natural high. Chilli is high in Vitamin C and has a range of health benefits, including fighting sinus congestion and aiding digestion. Chilli is also known to be a metabolism booster.

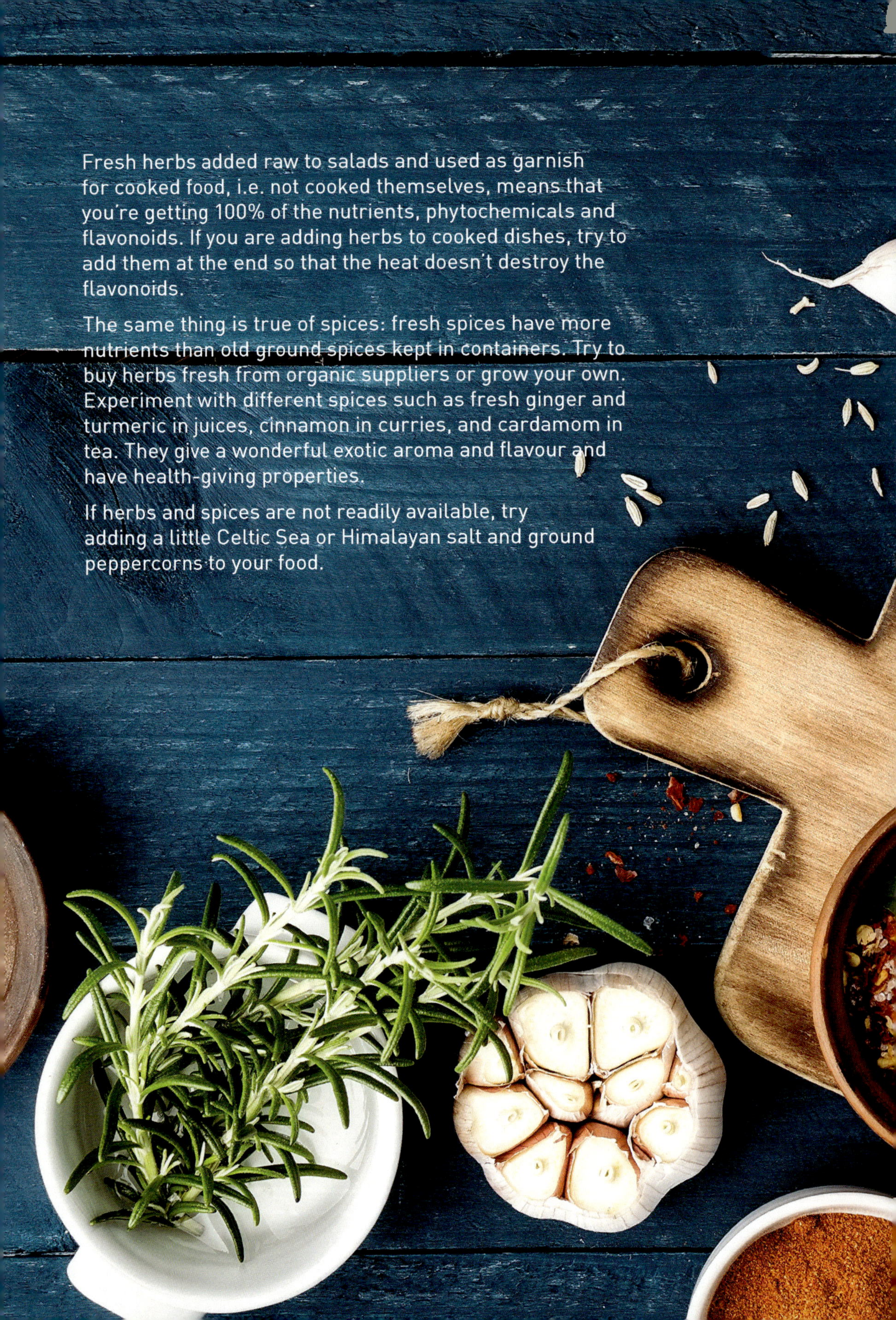

Fresh herbs added raw to salads and used as garnish for cooked food, i.e. not cooked themselves, means that you're getting 100% of the nutrients, phytochemicals and flavonoids. If you are adding herbs to cooked dishes, try to add them at the end so that the heat doesn't destroy the flavonoids.

The same thing is true of spices: fresh spices have more nutrients than old ground spices kept in containers. Try to buy herbs fresh from organic suppliers or grow your own. Experiment with different spices such as fresh ginger and turmeric in juices, cinnamon in curries, and cardamom in tea. They give a wonderful exotic aroma and flavour and have health-giving properties.

If herbs and spices are not readily available, try adding a little Celtic Sea or Himalayan salt and ground peppercorns to your food.

Conversion charts

Oven temperatures

Celsius (electric)	Celcius (fan forced)	Fahrenheit	Gas	
120°	100°	250°	1	Very slow
150°	130°	300°	2	Slow
160°	140°	325°	3	Moderately slow
180°	160°	350°	4	Moderate
190°	170°	375°	5	Moderately hot
200°	180°	400°	6	Hot
230°	210°	450°	7	Very hot
250°	230°	500°	9	Very hot

If using a fan-forced oven, your cooking time may be a little quicker, so start checking your food earlier.

Metric cup and spoon sizes

Cup	Metric
¼ cup	60ml
⅓ cup	80ml
½ cup	125ml
1 cup	250ml
Spoon	**Metric**
¼ teaspoon	1.25ml
½ teaspoon	2.5ml
1 teaspoon	5ml
2 teaspoons	10ml
1 tablespoon (equal to 4 teaspoons)	20ml

Liquid

Metric	Cup	Imperial
60ml	¼ cup	2 fl oz
80ml	⅓ cup	2 ¾ fl oz
125ml	½ cup	4 fl oz
180ml	¾ cup	6 fl oz
250ml	1 cup	8 ¾ fl oz
310ml	1 ¼ cups	10 ½ fl oz
375ml	1 ½ cups	13 fl oz
430ml	1 ¾ cups	15 fl oz
500ml	2 cups	17 fl oz
625ml	2 ½ cups	21 ½ fl oz
750ml	3 cups	26 fl oz
1L	4 cups	35 fl oz
1 ¼L	5 cups	44 fl oz
1 ½L	6 cups	52 fl oz
2L	8 cups	70 fl oz
2 ½L	10 cups	88 fl oz

Dry

Metric	Imperial
10g	¼ oz
15g	1/2oz
30g	1oz
60g	2oz
125g	4oz (¼ lb)
185g	6oz
250g	8oz (½ lb)
375g	12oz (¾ lb)
440g	14oz
500g (½ kg)	16oz (1 lb)
1kg	32oz (2 lb)

General portions table

	Serve size	Approx. serves per day FOR KIDS	Female	Male
CARBOHYDRATES		4		
Bread	1 slice	1-2	1 slice	2 slices
Cereal	¾ cup	1	½ cup	1 cup
Rice	½ cup	1	½ cup	1 cup
FRUIT &VEG				
Vegetables	80g	5	80g	100g
Apple/OTHER	Small apple	1-2	Small apple	Medium apple
PROTEIN		2		
Chicken	100g	1	100g	200g
Eggs	2 small eggs	1	1 large	2 large
DAIRY		2		
Cheese	2 slices	1	40g	40g
Yoghurt	½ cup	1	½ cup	¾ cup

Example for a child

Breakfast: cereal with milk and berries (1 carb + 1 dairy + 1 fruit)

Morning tea: 1 banana (1 fruit)

Lunch: sandwich with chicken and salad (1 protein + 2 carb + 1 veg)

Snack: cheese and crackers + carrot sticks + cucumber sticks (1 dairy + 1 veg)

Dinner: fish with boiled rice and mixed vegetables (1 protein + 1 carb + 3 vegetables)

Note: protein is also found in dairy foods such as milk, cheese and yoghurt.

NOTE

These are recommendations only. As children grow and participate in more activity/sport, their needs for energy and protein will change. Check with your nutrition coach for their specific requirements.

#Just eat real food!

From my experience we all think we eat well, but after 25 years of consultations I find this is simply not the case.

Let's be honest: There are times when I don't eat well or I indulge, but this is not on a daily basis.

When I see supermarket trolleys full of food, I often wonder if that would be the case if I could have just 30 minutes of their time, put back the packaged processed foods and show them how easy it is to eat real food.

We should be eating less from a box or packet and more natural foods that come from the land or are in their natural state. For example, let's take breakfast cereal in a box, which is often high in salt and sugars. You can make your own with nuts, seeds, cinnamon, activated buckwheat and coconut. It will taste great and be much healthier for you!

There are always better food choices.

Our App which is available on the App store has approved products by supermarket category to help you make better choices and to start moving in the right direction – one step at a time.

It's not always easy for us to cook from scratch and it's OK occasionally to take the easier option, but try not to do it too often.

Today the supermarket does give us options – there are pre-cut vegetables, marinated proteins and salad bags from which you can make a quick, nutritious meal.

I find that educating my clients with options and ideas makes it easier for them to make changes towards a healthy balanced life. There is nothing we cannot work with. A work routine or travelling? We have you covered!

Alongside choice of food comes portion size, water, food preparation, sugar, carbohydrates, fats and fads. Once these topics are explained, people have a much better understanding of what foods to combine, how much is needed, and how to prepare them.

While a nutrition consultation is overwhelming for some, we make it simple, non-clinical, and easy for you to create new habits and make the necessary changes to fit in with your lifestyle.

Our role is to bring passion, simplicity and sustainability into everyday life.

Useful references

The Food Coach Institute

Australia	www.iahnc.com
International	www.healthandnutritioncoaches.com
Facebook	www.facebook.com/TheFoodCoachInstitute

Foodfix4life

www.foodfix4life.com.au

Facebook	www.facebook.com/foodfix4life
App	foodfix4life.com.au/food-fix-4-life-app
Instagram	www.instagram.com/foodfix4life

Stop. Get Ready. Go.

Our first book is available on our website www.shop.foodfix4life.com.au

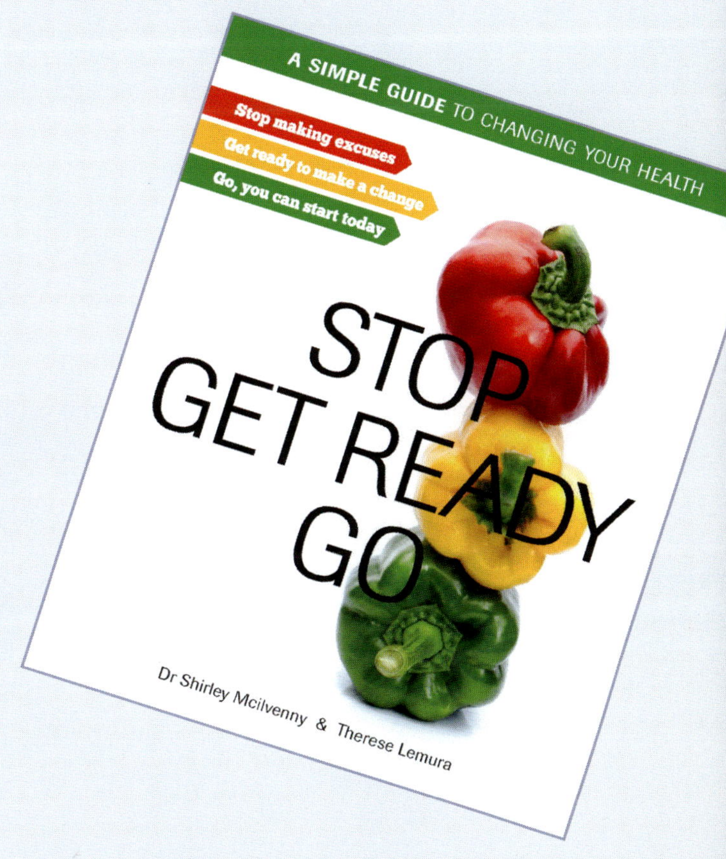

Q & A with Therese & Shirley

What is your favourite food and drink?

T – Ice cream and coffee.

S – Avocado and champagne.

Do you practise what you preach?

T – Yes. I eat well most of the time and exercise three to four times a week.

S – Yes, most of the time. We all have our bad days when we react to stress and then pig out but if you listen to your body, it will tell you what it needs.

How do you relax?

T – With a good cup of coffee.

S – Reading a good book.

What could you not live without?

T – My girls, Isabella and Liana.

S – Apart from my family – a good challenge.

How did you meet?

T – I did two of Shirley's courses through her institute.

S – Student and teacher got on like a house on fire.

Who inspires you?

T – Athletes.

S – Innovators and those who challenge the status quo.

Favourite female/male artist?

T – Tina Arena and Michael Bublé.

S – Pink and Andrea Bocelli.

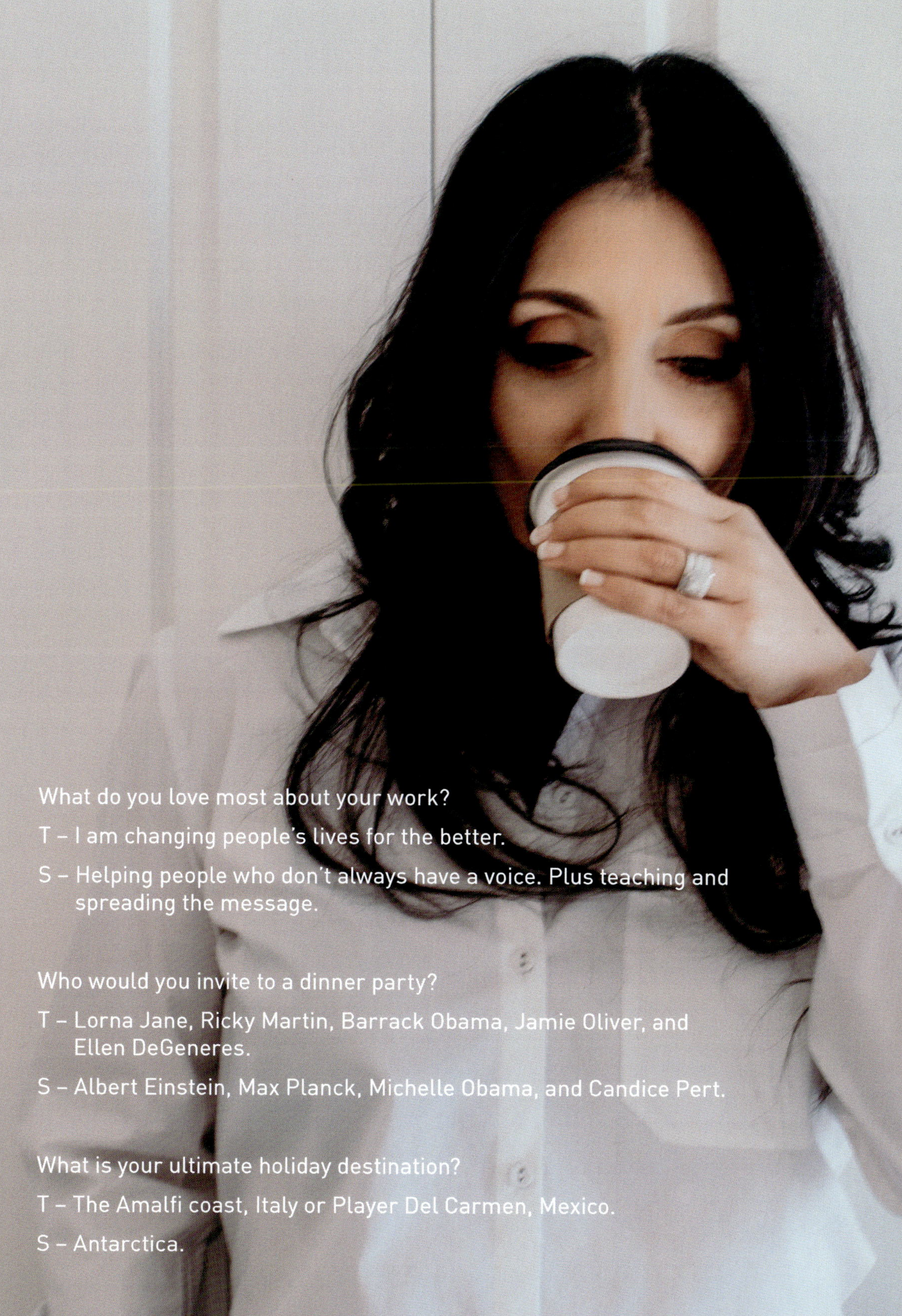

What do you love most about your work?

T – I am changing people's lives for the better.

S – Helping people who don't always have a voice. Plus teaching and spreading the message.

Who would you invite to a dinner party?

T – Lorna Jane, Ricky Martin, Barrack Obama, Jamie Oliver, and Ellen DeGeneres.

S – Albert Einstein, Max Planck, Michelle Obama, and Candice Pert.

What is your ultimate holiday destination?

T – The Amalfi coast, Italy or Player Del Carmen, Mexico.

S – Antarctica.

Balance and Perspective

Finding what works for you is the key to long-term sustainability. We are not all the same, so what works for some may not work for you. Most of us do not have chefs to prepare our meals, personal trainers to exercise with, babysitters to look after our children, or cleaners to clean our houses. When we are working, running a household, and running after the kids, finding a balance can be difficult.

Is change easy? Not for everybody, so embark on the health journey when you are truly ready. Do it for yourself and no one else. Start with just a few changes at a time; this will ensure all the everyday things such as work, kids, and cleaning are still being attended to.

Put your own situation under the perspective microscope. Remember, what other people can fit into a day may not be realistic or even easy for you to think about right now.

Sit down, assess your current situation regarding your commitments, surroundings, and motivation, and commit to making one meal change and one movement change a day.

One home-cooked meal instead of three take-away meals a day is definitely a step in the right direction. Use the night prior to prepare and chop your food, and before you know it those three take-away meals become one, because dinner and breakfast is planned and pre-prepared. Yes, planning is the key!

Walk to the shops three times a week instead of driving. An early-morning walk three times a week before the kids wake up is an achievable movement change.

Every day will not be the same, so adjust and compromise when necessary.

When a small change becomes routine, you start to see results and will of course feel better for it. Realistically balance your likes and dislikes every day with better time management, better food choices, a little exercise, and some downtime.

Need help with cooking? Try our recipes first; they are quick, easy and practical! There are many online places that deliver either cooked or fresh ingredient boxes for all your weekly meals.

TIP

Have you tried ordering fresh organic produce online? What about taking a drive to an organic farm and buying directly from them? It saves time, lasts longer, and tastes great!

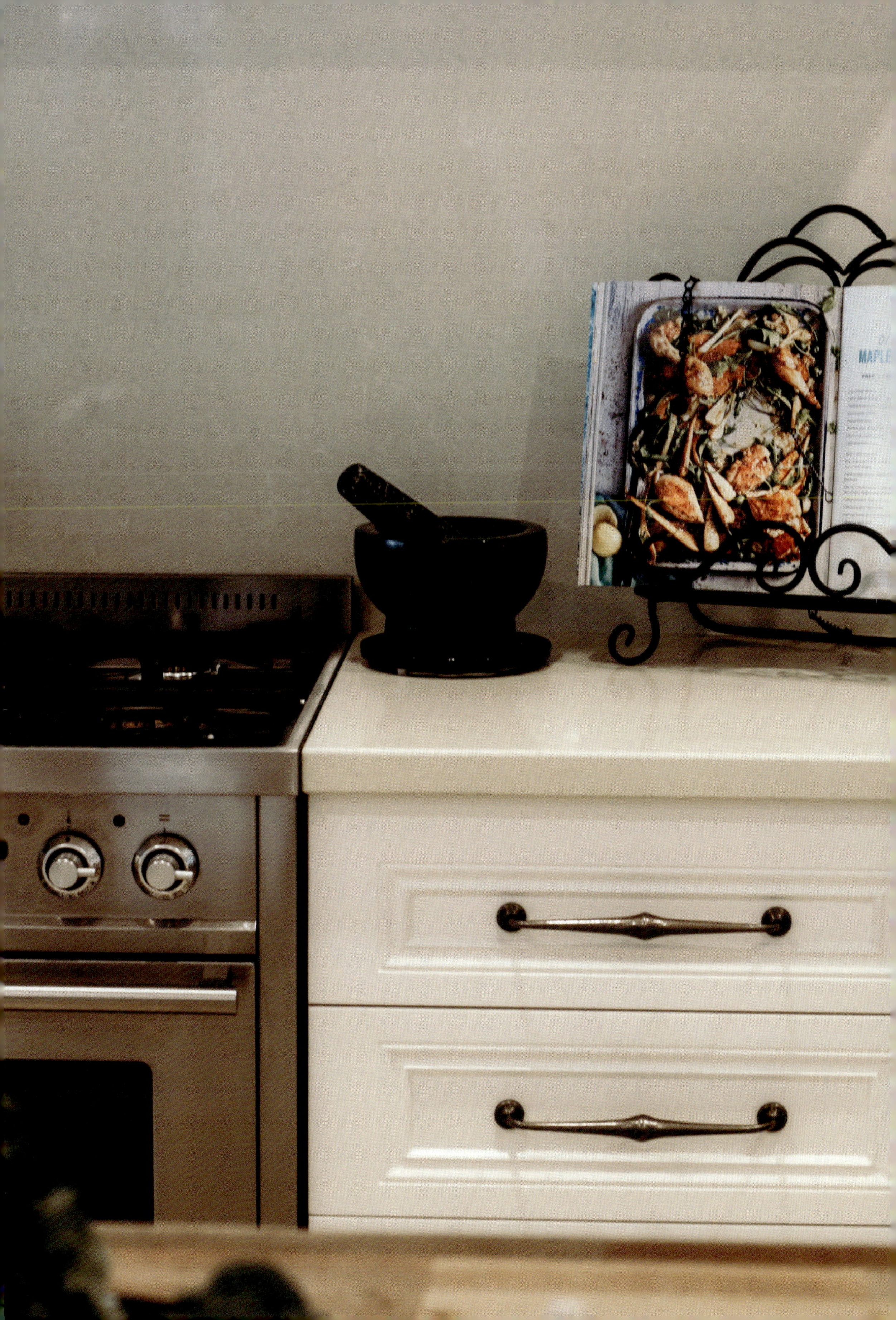
MAPLE

Summary

Being a parent and raising children has its challenges. The underlying message of this book is to produce healthy children, you need to teach them good eating and exercise habits at a young age. Say no, be firm, and remember the 80/20 rule so kids can be kids.

A parent constantly educating and leading by example will set great foundations with food and health. It will, in time, ensure our kids can make the right choices and decisions for themselves.

We hope this book has covered many aspects of good nutrition that you will find useful to use each day. Good health is not a short-term plan: It is a commitment for life. Incorporating our suggested foods and lifestyle tips will help you nourish your family. We understand not every day will be perfect as situations arise beyond our control, that's life, and we just pick up where we left off.

Be it weight loss, maintenance or just good health, factors such as stress, sleep, metabolic rate, and thyroid conditions need constant attention and care. A balanced lifestyle with sensible eating, and no fad dieting is the way to go.

Kids thrive on routine and consistency. When routine becomes habit, we see results that are sustainable.

There is so much information available on being healthy. We suggest you find what works for you, and be mindful of the media and non-reputable sites.

Eat well, feel well, live well. These words are progressive and truly promote a happy, balanced lifestyle.

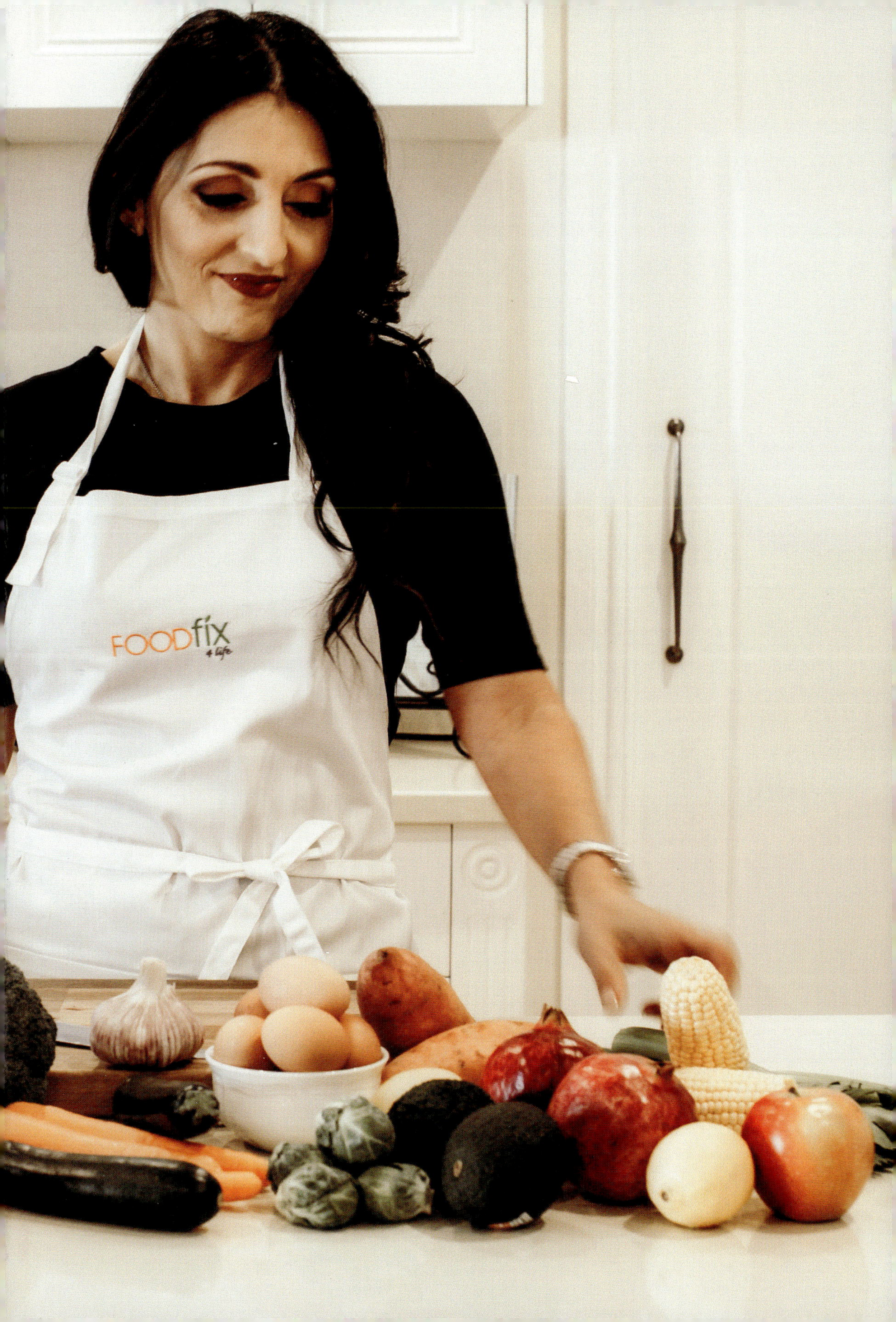
FOODfix
4 life

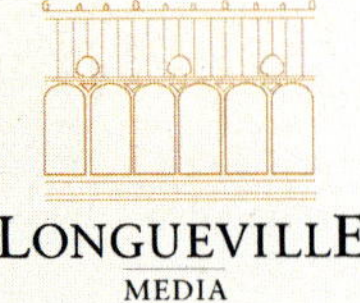

First published 2019
for Therese Lemura and Shirley Mcilvenny
by
Longueville Media Pty Ltd
PO Box 205 Haberfield NSW 2045 Australia
www.longmedia.com.au
info@longmedia.com.au
T. +61 410 519 685

Print PB ISBN: 978-0-6485107-7-2
Print HB ISBN: 978-0-6486978-3-1

A catalogue entry for this book is available from the National Library of Australia.